Ph

MW01491293

Improving M....... .....   ᴗ

Clinical Pharmacy Pearls,
Case Studies, & Common Sense

Eric Christianson, Pharm.D., BCPS, CGP
Edited by: Alissa Grimes, Pharm.D., BCPS

Copyright and Disclaimer

Cover Illustration and Design Copyright 2015 by: Melissa Christianson

Editing by: Alissa Grimes Pharm.D., BCPS

Formatting by: Melissa Christianson

ABOUT THE AUTHOR

Eric Christianson, Pharm.D., BCPS, CGP is a clinical pharmacist who is passionate about patient safety. Eric is the founder of meded101.com, a website dedicated to providing quality, free, real world medication education for healthcare professionals. He has been quoted or acknowledged by The Wall Street Journal, American Journal of Nursing, National Association Directors of Nursing, Pharmacy Podcast, Pharmacy Today, and Pharmacy Times.

Please take the time to check out the free resources provided through the website and social media accounts.

Free 6 page PDF at meded101.com - 30 Medication Mistakes

Facebook – https://www.facebook.com/meded101

Twitter - @mededucation101

LinkedIn – Eric Christianson, Pharm.D., BCPS, CGP

INTRODUCTION

Medication management gets more challenging every day. I created this resource to improve patient safety. Throughout the book, I provide real world scenarios to help you develop your medication common sense. I also educate healthcare professionals about some of the mistakes that I've seen in my everyday practice as a clinical pharmacist. I hope you enjoy the cases, short stories, and clinical pearls throughout the book.

Please feel free to reach out to me at mededucation101@gmail.com. You may also contact me through my website at https://www.meded101.com, where you can also find regularly updated, free medication education.

Table of Contents

CASE STUDIES

Lamotrigine (Lamictal) Rash

A patient had a seizure thought to be due to not taking their alprazolam (Xanax) over a period of a few days and was hospitalized as a result. The individual apparently had a seizure history in the past, but this was not clear in the medical records. During the hospitalization, it was noted that she had been on lamotrigine 250 mg twice daily in the past and was not currently on any antiepileptic therapy. The patient was started back on this dose in the hospital to prevent future seizures. About 10 days later, the patient began to develop a rash on both arms. There is a boxed warning on lamotrigine that cautions against starting at too high of a dose or titrating the dose too quickly. In this case, the patient had been previously on the drug but had not taken it for a long time. If this is the case, remember to start the titration over. Lamotrigine has a very slow titration process due to the risk of rash/Stevens-Johnson Syndrome which can potentially be life threatening. With this situation, the drug was inappropriately restarted at 20 times the normal dose! The recommended starting dose is 25 mg daily (dependent upon other medications being co-administered).

Anemia and Iron Supplementation

A common issue with surgery is post-op anemia due to blood loss during the procedure. A patient's hemoglobin dropped from 12.5 to 9.8 mg/dl, and the prescriber wanted to improve the hemoglobin back to baseline. Iron is a necessary component in the formation of red blood cells and is often supplemented following blood loss to ensure adequate iron stores for red blood cell production. This particular patient was told to go pick up some iron at the pharmacy and take it twice daily. The patient did just what he was told and continued to take the iron indefinitely even though he did not require iron before the surgery. Upon yearly hemoglobin checks, the patient certainly was not anemic. In this patient, long-term iron was not necessary as dietary intake was adequate, anemia had resolved via CBC checks, and the patient had no clinical symptoms. Iron supplementation should've been reassessed and discontinued much sooner, saving on potential drug interactions, side effects, and financial considerations, but the patient was simply doing what he was told.

Spironolactone (Aldactone) Induced Hyperkalemia

Often in CHF, you may see spironolactone used in combination with loops and other diuretics to try to help treat edema. There are certainly other indications for spironolactone, but I'll leave that for another case. My patient was having difficulty with edema, and increasing the loop diuretic was not improving the symptoms. Spironolactone was added to try to augment the fluid loss and improve CHF symptoms. Spironolactone is a potassium sparing diuretic and therefore raises potassium levels in the body, which is opposite from loop and thiazide diuretics which deplete potassium. This patient already had a potassium level around 4.8 mEq/L prior to the addition of the spironolactone (normal range 3.5 to 5.0 mEq/L). A couple weeks after initiating spironolactone, follow up electrolytes were drawn, and the potassium level was 5.9 mEq/L, necessitating the discontinuation of spironolactone. Bottom line, spironolactone can increase potassium levels, and keep a really close eye on those patients whose baseline level is already near the upper limit of normal when initiating or increasing spironolactone.

Escitalopram (Lexapro) Case and Antipsychotic Use

I had a resident at a nursing home that was prescribed escitalopram for depressive and anxiety symptoms. A few weeks after starting this medication, the resident developed worsening confusion, a change in cognition, and was physically and verbally aggressive with staff. It was apparent that something was going on. The antipsychotic quetiapine (Seroquel) was ordered to try to help with the delirium and aggressive behaviors. Escitalopram was continued for a few more days, and labs were ordered to try to decipher what caused the patient's change in status. Labs revealed that the resident had hyponatremia (low sodium) which can be caused by SSRI's like escitalopram. Escitalopram was discontinued, the low sodium resolved, and the resident improved. I can't stress enough the importance of trying to avoid the use of other medications (i.e. quetiapine in this case) to treat side effects of other medications! This is a classic example of the prescribing cascade. The prescribing cascade is one of my Top 30 Medication Mistakes – a free resource for subscribers at meded101.com.

Statin Induced Myopathy

A patient was admitted for a rehab stay at a long term care facility. The chief complaint was weakness and muscle achiness that would not resolve. While looking back at the patient history and medication list, it was clear that nothing was helping this patient. She did not have a fever, and various infections had been ruled out several times. Testing for less common diseases like Lyme's and West Nile were considered and ruled out as well. What was surprising (but not that surprising as she was on 30+ medications) to me was that this patient was on the highest recommended dose of atorvastatin (Lipitor), 80 mg daily, and this was never ruled out as the potential cause. Unfortunately, I was not able to follow up with this particular patient to find out if the statin was contributing to the myopathy symptoms, but it brings me to the point that when a patient is on a bunch of medications, medication side effects should be our first consideration when identifying a new complaint or concern.

The Diuretic Effect

An 81 year old gentleman was struggling with CHF symptoms. Fluid overload was the major problem causing significant difficulty with breathing. His furosemide (Lasix) was increased from 20 mg daily up to 40 mg daily to help promote the loss of fluid. Three days later, the increase in furosemide did not have a great enough effect, and metolazone (Zaroxolyn) 5 mg daily was added to augment the fluid loss. The provider ordered a follow up BMP to assess electrolytes and creatinine two weeks after starting the metolazone prescription.

The baseline potassium level was about 3.5 to 3.7 mEq/L prior to the increase in furosemide and addition of metolazone. At the two week check, the potassium was down to a critical low of 2.4 mEq/L. This case is just a simple reminder that there is a reason why lab monitoring is necessary, and patients can run into serious problems very quickly if not kept a close eye on, especially when significant changes are made. Dosing and frequency of these changes can make a huge difference in how aggressive we get in lab monitoring.

Drug Induced Edema

A 64 year old male patient was struggling with blood pressure management, usually running in the 160's range (systolic). He was already taking lisinopril (Zestril) 40 mg daily and had failed at implementing lifestyle changes up to this point. Nifedipine extended release (Procardia) 30 mg daily was added to this patient's regimen. It had minimal effect on the patient's blood pressure, and the dose was slowly titrated up to 120 mg daily. This dropped the systolic blood pressure 10-20 points on average, but the patient refused to continue to take the medication due to bothersome edema. This patient was successfully transitioned to a beta-blocker as well as a low dose thiazide diuretic for blood pressure management. Calcium channel blockers are effective at lowering blood pressure, but they are also one of the most common medication causes of edema especially at higher doses.

Phenytoin (Dilantin) Can Cause Vitamin D Deficiency

Phenytoin is probably one of the dirtiest drugs on the market, but can be necessary as it treats an obviously serious condition (seizures). It has many clinical quirks that you need to be aware of. A 72 year old female with a long history of seizures was on a maintenance dose of 200 mg twice daily. Seizures were well managed, and the patient displayed no symptoms of phenytoin toxicity with a total phenytoin level of 12. This particular patient was recently admitted to the hospital for a wrist fracture and subsequently diagnosed with osteoporosis. Upon this discovery, the provider ordered a vitamin D level to assess if/how much supplementation was necessary. The level came back at 6 nmol/L (normal is 30-100 in most labs). Why was this level so low? Long term phenytoin can cause/worsen vitamin D deficiency. The patient was started on a vitamin D supplement.

Bupropion (Wellbutrin) and Seizure Risk

A 69 year old male had significant respiratory issues including COPD. This patient was challenging but did have the intent to quit smoking which was certainly complicating his respiratory status. Other chronic conditions included: Coronary Artery Disease, Hypertension, Hypercholesterolemia, Seizures, and GERD. He had been displaying signs/symptoms of depression, and the primary physician decided to start bupropion extended release 150 mg daily with the idea of helping the depression. Bupropion can also have the added benefit of potentially helping with smoking cessation. After one week, a dose increase was made to 300 mg daily. On about day 10 since first initiating the bupropion, the patient had a seizure. He had previously been very well controlled; it had been at least a year since his last seizure. It is very important to remember that bupropion is well known for lowering seizure threshold (i.e. can increase the risk of seizures). It made perfect sense to start this medication for the duplicate role of smoking cessation and depressive symptoms, but the risk of bupropion lowering seizure threshold was overlooked.

Chemotherapy Induced Neuropathy

A 68 y/o male was undergoing chemotherapy treatments. As you may know, neuropathy can be a common side effect of certain chemo medications. This gentleman was battling through constant neuropathy type pain and was initiated on gabapentin (Neurontin) 300 mg twice daily. In this case of chemotherapy induced neuropathy, this dose was tolerated without issue, and chemotherapy cycles continued as scheduled with excellent results.

Following his chemo treatments, this patient ended up in remission upon rechecks with his oncologist. However, the gabapentin stayed on board even as this patient's symptoms of neuropathy resolved. Remembering to address ongoing medication use at every visit is an important aspect in the goal of preventing polypharmacy. It is one of my 10 Commandments of Polypharmacy. This is a case where it didn't happen. Sometimes the neuropathy can linger, but we need to continually reassess indefinite use of all medications.

Magnesium in Chronic Kidney Disease

A 78 year old male was receiving chronic opioid therapy for back pain as well as acetaminophen/diphenhydramine (Tylenol PM) one tablet at bedtime for sleep. This gentleman had been struggling with constipation issues and had been taking docusate (Colace) 100 mg daily for prevention.

This was not working well enough for him, so he started to take Milk of Magnesia 30 ml every day which did help with constipation. He continued to take this for weeks as any patient most likely would since it was beneficial for him. With a creatinine clearance around 25 ml/min, this patient was fortunate to have a routine check of labs which happened to include a magnesium level. Upon checking his magnesium, he was asymptomatic, but it was significantly elevated at 2.5 mEq/L (normal range of 1.2-1.9 depending upon lab). The educational point here is that magnesium can accumulate in chronic kidney disease, and education of our patients is extremely important! The use of magnesium in chronic kidney disease can be seemingly innocent but can have substantially negative side effects when given to the wrong patient.

Are you enjoying this content? If so, you'd be doing me a huge favor if you'd leave a star rating and review on Amazon where you purchased the book! Thanks in advance!

Diabetes Case – Canagliflozin (Invokana)

In making some of these decisions about medication changes, there isn't always a perfect answer. Caring professionals will disagree with one another. A nursing home resident was started on canagliflozin. He was also on a moderate dose of insulin glargine (Lantus) – about 30-40 units daily if I recall right. The provider did feel that blood sugars had improved a few months after initiation of canagliflozin. The A1C results told a different story. The A1C went from 8.2 to 8.1% three months later. So, would this justify the argument to continue a drug that's in the ballpark of 300$/month? For me, I'd prefer to increase the insulin (with no recent low blood sugars or signs of hypoglycemia) versus continuing with the canagliflozin. This is a bit of an oversimplification, but I think this case demonstrates that there is "more than one way to skin a cat" as my gruff former high school science teacher would say!

Pioglitazone (Actos) and CHF

A patient's A1C was chronically high at around 9.0% with poor diet compliance. She was already receiving a fairly high dose of a sulfonylurea (glipizide) and metformin 1,000 mg twice daily. Being on higher doses of two oral antidiabetic medications and still not having very good control, some might make the argument that insulin would be the next step. I would probably tend to agree with that in another case similar to this, but we have to treat people, not numbers. This patient would not take an injection no matter what, so the provider decided to add pioglitazone to try to lower the A1C without adding an injection. Sugars improved only mildly, but what was of note is that this patient had congestive heart failure. The patient's heart failure symptoms worsened following addition of the pioglitazone. It was discontinued, heart failure symptoms improved, and a DPP-4 inhibitor was initiated to help with diabetes management.

NSAIDs and GI Bleeding

A patient was having difficulty with symptoms of gout. He was on allopurinol 300 mg daily for hyperuricemia (elevated uric acid happens in gout). This patient would have flares periodically and had about three over the last year requiring the use of indomethacin 50 mg three times daily for up to a week at times. Due to ongoing issues with these gout flares and trials of multiple different medications for gout, the prescriber wrote for the patient to have an order for the indomethacin as needed without a limit on the length of use. Indomethacin is notorious for causing GI bleeding but is also a hallmark medication for the symptomatic treatment of a gout flare. In this case, the patient experienced great relief from the indomethacin 50 mg three times daily, but without the limit on how long the patient should use it, he continued use indefinitely. Within a couple weeks of consistent use of the indomethacin, the elderly gentleman was hospitalized, experiencing significant GI distress and black tarry stools indicating the presence of an NSAID induced ulcer. Often if chronic NSAID therapy is required, prescribers will use GI protection (usually a PPI such as omeprazole or pantoprazole or an H2 blocker like famotidine or ranitidine). In this case, the patient was not on GI protection and ended up with a GI bleed and hospital stay as a result.

Sertraline (Zoloft) and Loose Stools

A 57 year old patient diagnosed with depression was initiated on sertraline 50 mg daily. The physician in this case felt that the patient was very depressed and wanted to titrate the dose up fairly quickly. Sertraline was increased to 100 mg daily after two weeks and then further to 150 mg two weeks after that. Remember that patient adherence to medications (especially antidepressant therapy) can be challenging due to the fact that most patients are not going to experience any relief in their depressive symptoms on a short term basis. However, the side effects from antidepressant therapy can be apparent immediately upon starting the medication. A couple days after the increase to 100 mg daily, the patient began experiencing troubling loose stools occurring multiple times per day. Patients are usually very perceptive to the side effects of medications, especially when the initiation of the medication and the onset of the side effects correlate. This patient ended up stopping the sertraline on his own due to the intolerable side effects and refused further antidepressant therapy.

Amoxicillin Allergy or Something Else

I really want to encourage younger healthcare professionals to ask questions and realize that no matter how experienced you are, there are going to be times throughout your career where you don't know an answer. There will also be times where caring professionals disagree.

Case Study:
Day 1: An 18 month old boy on zero medications is diagnosed with a double ear infection and prescribed amoxicillin twice daily. He receives the first dose that evening.

Day 2-7: He has been taking amoxicillin as prescribed with zero missed doses. Symptoms of the ear infection have improved over this period.

Day 8: Mom notices a few spots (some about the size of a dime) all over different parts of the body. Because of this, the amoxicillin is held, and he is taken in for reassessment of rash and to assure ear infection has resolved. The last dose of amoxicillin was given on the eve of day 7. He is given a diagnosis of amoxicillin allergy. The ear infection appears mostly resolved so no further antibiotics are warranted, and amoxicillin is discontinued. Diphenhydramine (Benadryl) is recommended as needed for the rash, and it was anticipated that the rash would begin resolving upon discontinuing the amoxicillin. At this point, the boy has minimal rash on the face, no fever, and vitals are unremarkable.

Day 9: 18 month old sleeps through the night and wakes up looking much worse in the morning with extensive spreading of the rash. The right eye is nearly closed shut due to the soft tissue swelling around the eye.

Due to the worsening condition, an ER visit is made to assess the eye and worsening rash. Vitals and temperature are fine. Mood and appetite are relatively normal as well. Diagnosis is likely "classic" viral infection causing rash. The ER physician says there would be nearly zero doubt about the diagnosis had the patient not been on amoxicillin, but he believes it is a viral infection.

A visit to the regular pediatrician later that day leads to script for prednisolone. The primary pediatrician was non-committal on a diagnosis but thought it was hard to ignore the amoxicillin.

Day 10: With the use of diphenhydramine and prednisolone, the rash is fading and much less pronounced than day 9.

I tend to believe it was an allergic reaction. He had been around numerous other kids that week, so a contagious viral infection does also have some validity. This case demonstrates how caring healthcare professionals can and do disagree. So, what do you think? Was this an amoxicillin allergy, viral infection, combination, or something else? If you are in the camp of viral infection or something else, would you dare give amoxicillin again?

Antibiotic Failure: Iron and Levofloxacin (Levaquin) Drug Interaction

A 44 year old male with a history of asthma was recently diagnosed at the clinic with pneumonia. Levofloxacin was initiated for a 10 day period.

<u>Current Medications:</u>
Fluticasone/salmeterol (Advair) 250/50 twice daily
Albuterol as needed
Hydrochlorothiazide 25 mg daily
Ferrous sulfate 325 mg twice daily
Omeprazole (Prilosec) 20 mg daily

On Day 7 of 10 of the levofloxacin course, the patient is not improving. He presents to the clinic for reassessment of pneumonia and requests a different medication. Azithromycin (Zithromax/Zpak) is prescribed, and within 3-5 days, the patient begins feeling much better with a full resolution of the pneumonia following treatment with azithromycin.

So, what happened? We can only speculate, but I've got 3 major points that I think could've been the problem.

1. Assessment of adherence is critical with antibiotics and any medication for that matter – that is where I would start.
2. Resistance to antibiotics is a significant problem and could be at play here.
3. I've seen this happen several times, and I think it might lead to failure more often than we realize, especially with quinolone antibiotics. The iron and levofloxacin drug interaction is well known but does slip through the cracks, especially with polypharmacy complicating things. Iron can significantly block absorption of levofloxacin, leading to low concentrations in the blood that are

potentially low enough to cause failure of treatment. This is an interaction you should be aware of. We also need to assess for use of products containing iron, calcium, and magnesium which can all bind up quinolones.

Meet Midodrine, an Alpha Agonist

I had an elderly male patient started on midodrine due to symptomatic orthostasis. He was not receiving any other medications that would be likely to lower blood pressure.

This particular patient had a history of BPH which he was not currently on medication management for. The primary provider, noting worsening symptoms of retention following the addition of midodrine, added finasteride (Proscar) to help manage the symptoms. As you could imagine, the patient wasn't very happy with this as finasteride is a 5-alpha reductase inhibitor used to shrink the prostate. Per Lexicomp: "Clinical responses occur within 12 weeks to 6 months upon initiation of therapy".

With this brief scenario, I want to create two very important educational points.

1. Midodrine is an alpha agonist, and if we think about this mechanism of action, it directly opposes the action of alpha blockers commonly used for the acute (and sometimes long term) management of urinary retention usually due to BPH in males.
2. Lesson number two is a mistake I've seen a few times: the thought that finasteride or other 5 alpha reductase inhibitors (i.e. dutasteride) will treat BPH in the short term. As noted above, these drugs take a long time to work and are not going to provide relief short term.

An alternative option in this case would be fludrocortisone for orthostasis. This corticosteroid medication certainly has plenty of clinical quirks as well, so digging into the patient history would be critically important.

Drug Induced Hypertension Case

A 76 year old patient was on a laundry list of blood pressure medications including hydrochlorothiazide, losartan, metoprolol, terazosin, and amlodipine. Clonidine was also recently added to the regimen with minimal success. Systolic blood pressures still consistently ran around 160 even with aggressive treatment.

About a year ago, the patient was having really problematic pain associated with osteoarthritis and was self-treating with over-the-counter ibuprofen 600 mg (3 of the 200 mg tabs) three times daily. The patient had never tried acetaminophen (Tylenol) in the past. Many of the increases in blood pressure medications had come in the previous year. Point: NSAIDs can contribute/worsen high blood pressure, and in this case, the ibuprofen could've been ruled out sooner as the potential culprit. The patient was able to transition to acetaminophen, and the NSAID was discontinued. Systolic blood pressures improved to around 140-150 range.

Double Dose, Double Trouble – Phenytoin (Dilantin) Toxicity

A 98 y/o female with a long history of seizures was treated with phenytoin 100 mg twice daily. The phenytoin level was routinely drawn every 6 months and had been in the 6-10 mcg/ml range for quite some time (normal total level is

10-20 mcg/ml, but there are multiple variables that can make the value less than accurate). The most recent level was 5 mcg/ml, and the primary provider was concerned it was too low and increased the dose from 100 mg BID to 200 mg BID.

Keep in mind, this patient had not had a seizure for years. This patient's albumin was low as well, which actually increases the corrected phenytoin value. An increase in a maintenance dose like this with phenytoin should scare you. I have seen toxicity result several times due to inappropriate increases.

Phenytoin is metabolized by a few different enzymes, and when those enzymes get saturated, the amount of phenytoin in the body can skyrocket quickly. Think of a hockey stick type curve. So clinically what this means is that when you start to hit the upward slope of that curve, small increases in dose is the usual practice. MODERATE TO LARGE INCREASES IN PHENYTOIN DOSE CAN LEAD TO HUGE JUMPS IN LEVELS! Pharmacokinetics is an ugly word for some, but not knowing the kinetics of phenytoin can harm patients.

Within a week or two, this patient began displaying signs of phenytoin toxicity – GI symptoms, difficulty with walking, lethargy, and confusion. She was hospitalized and was diagnosed with phenytoin toxicity with a total level of 28 mcg/ml.

Serotonin Syndrome or Something Else?

An 88 y/o female who's had some difficulty with pain management was on scheduled acetaminophen (Tylenol) 1,000 mg twice daily as well as tramadol (Ultram) 50 mg every 6 hours as needed. She brought up the complaint about her osteoarthritis to her physician. She was then prescribed tramadol 100 mg four times daily scheduled. When I had spoken with the caregivers, they had been doing some research and were significantly concerned about serotonin syndrome due to increased confusion, general declining condition, and worsening mental status. This patient was also on an SSRI, citalopram (Celexa) 20 mg daily. There were no other symptoms of serotonin syndrome (tachycardia, elevated temp, etc.) besides the change in cognition. Serotonin syndrome is very serious, but the oversight in this case was that the patient was previously very reluctant to take the as needed tramadol. Upon discussion with caregivers, she was only taking the PRN tramadol one or two times daily on average. The increase from 50-100 mg per day to 400 mg per day was simply too aggressive in this case. Another key point is that the maximum recommended daily dose of tramadol is 300 mg for the elderly. Adverse effects improved with a reduction in the tramadol to 50 mg three times daily.

Pseudoephedrine (Sudafed) Side Effects and the Prescribing Cascade

An 89 year old patient has been battling with anxiety and insomnia over the previous few months. The past medical history also includes GERD, hypertension, allergies/congestion, and constipation.

Current Medications:
Lorazepam 0.25 mg twice daily as needed
Diphenhydramine 25 mg daily at bedtime
Omeprazole 20 mg daily
Lisinopril 20 mg daily
Metoprolol 25 mg twice daily

Hydrochlorothiazide 25 mg daily
Pseudoephedrine 60 mg every 4-6 hours as needed
Clonidine 0.1 mg twice daily
Docusate 100 mg twice daily
Senna 2 tablets twice daily

The first thing I would look at addressing is the current problem. With anxiety and insomnia, I'd be concerned that the pseudoephedrine side effects are exacerbating these conditions and causing potentially unnecessary use of other medications. Timing is very important as always. Is he taking the pseudoephedrine, how often, and when did he start taking it? I'd also look and see if any of the blood pressure medications have been increased with the timing of the pseudoephedrine.

We also have some issues with constipation. This is a perfect example of the potential of the prescribing cascade. Is pseudoephedrine worsening hypertension, causing the use of more blood pressure medications? Is it causing insomnia, necessitating the use of the diphenhydramine? Is it causing or worsening anxiety and inciting the use of lorazepam? Is the diphenhydramine causing the use of the laxatives (docusate and Senna)? Just a few thoughts on the importance of assessing as needed medication use.

Amiodarone and Thyroid Function

An 88 year old with a history of depressive type symptoms was placed on an antidepressant shortly after admission to a long term care facility.

This patient was trialed on sertraline (Zoloft) and then transitioned to duloxetine (Cymbalta), neither of which made a significant difference in symptoms. This patient continued to have ongoing symptoms of depression despite antidepressant therapy.

Hypothyroid symptoms can often overlap/mimic signs of depression, and this is a scenario I've seen play out several times. What was of note was that the patient was on chronic amiodarone for an arrhythmia. Amiodarone has many unique side effects, one of which is it can affect thyroid function. It was requested that a TSH be checked to monitor for this unique side effect of amiodarone, and the TSH results were elevated at about 30 indicating hypothyroidism (normal range is approximately 0.5-6 depending upon the lab). Levothyroxine (Synthroid) was initiated and the symptoms of "depression" started to improve, allowing for discontinuation of the duloxetine.

What Does too Much Levothyroxine (Synthroid) Look Like?

I had a long term care resident that was experiencing anxiety, tachycardia, weight loss, and was a nightmare as far as trying to manage behavioral issues. I had discussed the resident's situation with the nursing staff, and they weren't exactly sure what was going on. The provider had started the resident on an SSRI (frequently used for anxiety disorders) and added a dose of lorazepam as needed to help treat the symptoms.

While reviewing the chart, I noted that the TSH was low and the resident was on levothyroxine 88 mcg daily. This would seem to indicate that the resident had too high of a dose. The low level was noted and the provider inadvertently increased the dose to 100 mcg daily, actually worsening the suppression of TSH. The dosing of levothyroxine based on TSH is counter intuitive; when

TSH is elevated, it generally indicates hypothyroidism, and a low TSH notes too much supplementation or hyperthyroidism. Fast forward a few months later after the dose was appropriately reduced to 75 mcg daily: The TSH had returned to normal limits, and the anxiety symptoms had improved. The SSRI and lorazepam were able to be discontinued as well.

Falls in the Elderly

An 84 year old female suffers from frequent falls, CAD, atrial fibrillation, CHF, anxiety, dementia (including frequently yelling out at night), constipation and diabetes.

Current Medications
Warfarin 2.5 mg daily
Meclizine 25 mg q 4hr as needed
Valsartan 320 mg daily
Metoprolol 50 mg twice daily
Furosemide 40 mg daily
Alprazolam 1 mg three times daily
Risperidone 0.5 mg at bedtime
Glipizide XL 5 mg daily

Falls in the elderly are incredibly challenging, and medications often contribute to that challenge. Here's a case where we have a patient who is frequently falling, and I want to highlight a few points that we need to be thinking about.

My first thought is the large dose of alprazolam. In general, this a steep dose, particularly for someone in their 80's. Meclizine prn also indicates to me that this patient is likely dizzy which could be from many of her medications.

We've got risk of orthostasis with blood pressure reducing medications as well as the risperidone. In addition, we don't have a good diagnosis for use of risperidone.

One thing that may get overlooked is the risk of hypoglycemia with the sulfonylurea – blood sugar monitoring will also be important when considering fall risk in this patient. When assessing falls in the elderly, it is critical to look at every medication!

With the obvious behavioral issues and dementia diagnosis, I'd like to further investigate the yelling at night and potentially rule out pain as a contributing factor. If this is the case, the risperidone and alprazolam could possibly be decreased or discontinued in the future. Another concern is that warfarin, or any blood thinner for that matter, could increase the risk of a life threatening bleed following a fall related injury.

DRUG INTERACTIONS

Drug Food Interactions

Two drug food interactions you need to know:

1. Statins (Zocor-simvastatin, Lipitor-atorvastatin, etc.) are some of the most widely used drugs in the US, and there is an interaction with grapefruit juice. Different clinicians tend to manage this in different ways, and management of this interaction should be done on a case by case basis. If a patient is adamant that they have grapefruit juice (I have seen them) – what do you do? Should a statin be stopped because of this? I don't believe so unless strong evidence exists that indicates potential for harm. The result from this interaction is that it increases the amount of the statin in the body. Lexicomp essentially states that if grapefruit juice will not be avoided, the patient should limit their intake to less than 7-10 ounces per day (about a cup). In my opinion, if you decide to continue to take grapefruit juice with the guidance of your pharmacist/doctor, small quantities are the way to go.

2. Vitamin K is essential for the formation of clotting factors and therefore essential for the formation of clots. It is widely found in various foods (i.e. green leafy vegetables, broccoli, asparagus, etc.). I've heard individuals say that vitamin K should be avoided if you are taking warfarin (Coumadin). This is simply not true. A variation in vitamin K intake can affect your INR however. It's important that patients be consistent in their vitamin K intake if they are on warfarin. More than the usual intake and your INR will likely drop. Take in less vitamin K than normal for a few days/weeks, and your INR will likely be higher.

Drug Interactions – When should we do something?

Is there really a standard way to deal with drug interactions? My answer: you cannot treat them all the same. I see all sorts of different faxes from different pharmacies as well as other healthcare programs in nursing homes, home cares, assisted livings, etc. warning of drug interactions. It's really just weird and a waste of time in many cases. I cannot recall one fax from a pharmacy or other institution about a patient taking an NSAID and warfarin. Not one, and trust me, I've seen these drugs used together numerous times. Maybe the individual looking at this assumes the prescriber is aware of this? This is a hallmark drug interaction and is on many top ten lists of the most concerning interactions, and I can't recall ever seeing a single fax?

The drug interaction fax I saw that really shocked me was the combination of an inhaled anticholinergic (ipratropium) with solid oral dosage forms of potassium. It was of the highest severity. The thought is that the anticholinergic effects slow GI motility, and the potassium can then cause ulceration or damage to the GI tract. Really??? I went to look up this interaction, and Lexicomp lists it as an "X" – the highest severity. Next, I looked up the amount absorbed into the body from inhaled ipratropium. It states "negligible". If systemic absorption is negligible, how is this an interaction, much less an interaction of highest severity? A computer program cannot provide common sense.

These programs are a tool, not a brain, and I do have a concern that some healthcare professionals may expect their programs to save them. We can all miss important interactions, and computer programs can help us flag interactions, but we need to give thoughtful clinical review of an interaction before dispensing, prescribing, or administering a medication.

Notes from Prescriber Letter article regarding Potassium/Inhaled Anticholinergics: "The interaction between potassium tablets and anticholinergic drugs has caused this problem (GI ulceration). Some (computer) systems apply this interaction to inhaled anticholinergic drugs, like tiotropium (Spiriva) or ipratropium (Atrovent). But, inhaled anticholinergic drugs act only in the lungs."

It's estimated that 330 drug interaction alerts have to be reviewed to prevent a single adverse drug reaction of any severity. To prevent a single serious adverse event, you would have to review more than 2700 alerts. To prevent a single event leading to death, disability or prolonged symptoms, you would need to review between 4200 and 44,000 alerts.

Source:
http://prescribersletter.therapeuticresearch.com/ce/cecourse.aspx?pc=12-216

Rifampin Drug Interaction

Rifampin is an enzyme inducer. What does this mean? Basically, rifampin causes enzymes in the body to chew up material (drugs, chemicals, etc.) more quickly. Changing this drug's dosing, starting the medication, or discontinuing the medication can change how drugs are metabolized. Starting the drug and changing the dose are generally no brainers as far as monitoring for interactions. What many people fail to remember is that discontinuing this drug can cause interaction problems as well. Here's a case example to demonstrate my point. A patient was placed on rifampin for osteomyelitis, an infection that generally takes a long time to treat. What ended up happening was that the warfarin (Coumadin) the individual was on needed to be escalated to above 15 mg per day because rifampin was increasing its clearance from the body. When this drug was stopped, it was inevitable that a surplus of warfarin would occur without a reduction in dose and close monitoring of the INR. The patient's INR was 2.1 and therefore at goal for atrial fibrillation shortly before rifampin was discontinued. After discontinuation, when the INR was rechecked 30 days later, it was dangerously high at 9.6.

Drug Interaction Causing Pregnancy

A 32 year old female had been struggling with fatigue, sadness, and overall symptoms of depression. Rather than utilizing traditional antidepressants as recommended by her primary care provider, the patient had heard from a friend that the herbal supplement St. John's Wort had helped with her symptoms, so she decided to give it a try. Three months later, the patient developed fatigue and had not had her normal monthly cycle. She took a pregnancy test and found out she indeed was expecting even though she had been taking her Ortho-Tri-Cyclen (birth control) as prescribed. What happened? We can never 100% say, but St. John's Wort does have the potential to reduce the effectiveness of birth control, making it more likely for an unanticipated pregnancy. St. John's Wort is a notorious herbal supplement that can interact with many prescription medications (cholesterol meds, seizure meds, warfarin, etc.). Even though there is easy access to herbal supplements and over-the-counter (OTC) medications, it does not always mean they are safe.

Case Study: Simvastatin and Diltiazem Interaction

A 66 year old female was newly diagnosed with atrial fibrillation. Her other diagnoses included hypertension, diabetes, hyperlipidemia, and GERD.

<u>Current Medications:</u>
Aspirin 81 mg daily
Simvastatin (Zocor) 40 mg at bedtime
Acetaminophen (Tylenol) as needed
Pantoprazole (Protonix) 40 mg daily
Lisinopril 10 mg daily
Metformin 500 mg twice daily

With the new diagnosis of atrial fibrillation, the primary provider started the patient on diltiazem (Cardizem) CD 180 mg daily.

Within a few weeks, the patient began to feel worsening muscle pains and aching. She could not attribute it to physical activity or anything else going on in her life. She began taking the acetaminophen as needed 2-3 times per day to try to help with the pain she was having.

Upon investigation of the medication regimen, it was discovered that the diltiazem had been started a few weeks back. Diltiazem can increase the serum concentration of simvastatin which is likely what happened in this case, leading to the muscle pain/soreness.

Per Lexicomp, simvastatin and diltiazem used together should be avoided if other alternatives exist. If use can't be avoided, a maximum recommended dose of simvastatin at 10 mg daily should be considered. The simvastatin and diltiazem interaction is one you need to be aware of!

Drug Interactions Checker – What's Relevant?

A computerized drug interactions checker can sometimes go way overboard leading to constant alerts that aren't taken seriously. We need better programs to help identify interactions, but more importantly, we need to develop the critical thinking skills to know how and when to address these alerts. In other words, we need to be able to figure out what's relevant.

I recently saw a drug interaction fax sent to the doctor about the risk of hyperkalemia when taking potassium and lisinopril (both low doses). The risk of this interaction was "severe" according to the computer report. So, is this really severe, and should a prescriber be alerted?

If the doses prescribed were unusually high, I could understand a heightened awareness, but there are other avenues to investigate this. This patient was also on furosemide (Lasix) and had a history of CHF. I'm a solution oriented individual, so instead of using the time to send that fax and have the doctor sign it (a fact they will know), maybe call and ask the clinic for the most recent potassium level or if lab work is planned in the near future. Another option would be to ask the patient if lab work is planned. They may or may not know, but engaging patients and making them active participants in their healthcare is always a good thing. The physician who had been practicing medicine for 10+ years (I would assume was insulted) refused to sign the fax. Everyone dispensing or prescribing should know that potassium supplements can elevate potassium. Don't get me wrong, dangerous potassium levels can result from ACE alone or in combination with potassium supplements, but a patient on a potassium supplement is going to have their potassium level checked. ACE inhibitors raise potassium, and so do potassium supplements. In my mind, this would be similar to alerting someone that adding aspirin to clopidogrel (Plavix) can increase bleed risk. If you do feel that you need to remind a prescriber about this "interaction", it might be appropriate to tell your patients they should see a different provider (kidding of course). Both examples should be common knowledge. This potassium interaction is monitored by checking lab work. In my opinion, simple things like this can really damage credibility amongst healthcare professionals. Additionally, when there is something potentially life threatening or harmful to address, is your voice going to be heard after sending seemingly meaningless information to the prescriber in the past?

Aspirin and Lisinopril Interaction

I was at a long term care facility and had a patient on lisinopril 10 mg daily for hypertension as well as aspirin 325 mg daily for cardiovascular prophylaxis. Lexicomp has the aspirin and lisinopril interaction rated at a C on a scale of A to D and X being contraindicated.

Putting myself in this situation, this is a great case where a solution could be offered rather than just notifying the physician. There are two solutions that initially come to my mind.

1. This patient was a resident of a long term care facility. The facility will have good information on the blood pressure results of this resident. The individual who was prompted with this interaction could certainly pick up the phone and inquire nursing staff about the blood pressure readings. Monitoring is so important when it comes to

drug interactions, and this option tends to slip through the cracks once in a while as I've seen some providers almost panic and not think about what the alert is actually saying.

2. The second solution would be to ask the provider to assess the current dose of aspirin. Per Lexicomp, this interaction doesn't occur or has minimal effect when the dose of aspirin is less than 100 mg daily. In many cases, we can get by with a dose of 81 mg daily.

Cimetidine and Drug Interactions

An 85 year old female with an extensive seizure history was on phenytoin (Dilantin) 300 mg daily. Previous phenytoin level was 14, and the patient was not displaying any signs or symptoms of toxicity. She began having some GI complaints and was diagnosed with GERD and placed on cimetidine. About 2 weeks later, it was noted that the nurses had described the resident as having a decline in status, increased confusion, difficulty walking, and increased sedation. A phenytoin level was eventually ordered. The total phenytoin level came back at 33! The healthcare team was very fortunate that it was caught soon enough before hospitalization or worse! Key point: cimetidine has several substantial drug interactions, and if you ever see it utilized, be sure you're not asleep at the wheel.

Levothyroxine (Synthroid) Interaction

I had a patient a while back struggling with ongoing depressive symptoms, fatigue, and constipation. Both mirtazapine (Remeron) and sertraline (Zoloft) had been tried without any benefit. The most recent TSH was elevated at 13, requiring an increase in the levothyroxine dose from 150 mcg to 175 mcg. Over the previous 6 months, the levothyroxine had been increased 3 different times from a previous dose of 100 mcg. About 10 months ago, the patient was diagnosed with osteoporosis and placed on a bisphosphate and calcium/vitamin D supplementation. The calcium was being administered at the same time as the levothyroxine and was preventing adequate absorption. With inadequate absorption, the dose had to be escalated from the patient's usual previous dose. Had the timing of the calcium been changed or timing of the levothyroxine been changed at the start of the calcium, the patient may have avoided the struggle of battling with hypothyroidism symptoms and two potentially unnecessary antidepressants. In a case like this, you may not see the effects of the calcium/levothyroxine interaction for a couple of months, and by that time, the addition of the calcium may have been long forgotten.

Fluvoxamine (Luvox) and Olanzapine (Zyprexa) Interaction

I had a resident in a nursing home who had an extensive psych history including episodes of physical aggression and schizophrenia. There also was also an element of obsessive-compulsive disorder (OCD). This patient was followed closely by psychiatry and was receiving a dose of olanzapine 15 mg at bedtime. To help with the OCD symptoms, the psychiatrist ordered the SSRI fluvoxamine which is rarely used due to the potential for multiple drug interactions. Within a few days upon initiation of the fluvoxamine, the patient was extremely lethargic and had a couple of falls. The most likely cause of this was an interaction where fluvoxamine significantly increases the blood levels of olanzapine, leading to potential toxicity. If you ever see an order for fluvoxamine, you must look for drug interactions!

CLINICAL PEARLS

Digoxin

Digoxin can be a challenging drug. If a patient is elderly, this can really complicate things. Another thing that can complicate digoxin dosing is renal function. Renal function usually declines with age, which can lead to the accumulation of many medications that are normally eliminated through the kidney. I've seen numerous cases of digoxin toxicity that show how easily digoxin can be overlooked. Usually the reason this slips through the cracks is because the patient on digoxin is generally on a boatload of other meds as well, creating confusion as to whether symptoms of toxicity are mimicking another disease process or are a side effect of a different medication. The aggressiveness of the dosing for digoxin can also vary depending upon the condition you are treating. Lower doses are usually utilized for heart failure. The classic case I've seen a handful of times: a patient has a decline in renal function, so less of the drug is eliminated and concentrations begin to rise in the body (pharmacokinetics matters!). Some signs and symptoms of digoxin toxicity include GI (nausea etc.), general confusion or change in cognition, weight loss, and low pulse. It's always important to look for "trigger" medications when trying to identify potential adverse effects. I consider "trigger" medications as those that mask potential adverse effects. In the case of digoxin, maybe you'd see promethazine or a PPI added for GI issues. I've also seen Alzheimer's medications such as memantine (Namenda) and donepezil (Aricept) added to help "treat" the confusion due to adverse effects.

Warfarin (Coumadin) Drug Interactions

Warfarin has a lot of drug interactions! This is one of the key traits of warfarin that makes it difficult to manage. One case I remember was an individual with dual infections going on; she was on fluconazole (Diflucan) for a fungal infection and trimethoprim/sulfamethoxazole (Bactrim) for a UTI. It had been a couple of days since they had started their courses of each of these, so an INR was requested. The INR came back greater than 10 (the lab wouldn't read it any higher than that). The higher the INR, the more "thin" the blood and hence the more likely you are to have a bleed. You may often hear that warfarin is a "blood thinner". Basically the moral of the story is anytime a drug is changed (increased, decreased, or discontinued) you have the potential to alter the levels of warfarin in the body. If you are not comfortable with common drug interactions, you need to look them up!

Metformin

Metformin is part of the biguanide class of diabetes meds – I don't know why I told you that because you will probably never need to know that, but I have been wrong before. Metformin is usually fairly well tolerated as long as we can avoid GI adverse effects. One of my pet peeves is when an elderly individual gets started on drugs that are notoriously bad for side effects and not tapered up slowly. I've seen cases where individuals get started on 1000 mg twice a day (a higher dose) and have GI side effects like nausea and loose stools. They then get taken off the drug, and it gets added to their intolerance list! Frustrating! They may not have tolerated it anyway, but now anyone will be hesitant to try it again, not knowing the background of the intolerance. In individuals with kidney disease, you want to take a close look to make sure this drug is appropriate as there is an elevated risk of lactic acidosis (very rare) in patients on metformin with poor kidney function.

Prednisone and Diabetes Management

In the case where an individual must be on a prednisone (or any other corticosteroid) burst, diabetes management can become challenging. A 78 year old patient with diabetes was fairly well managed. Her A1C was hovering in the 7 range or lower. She was on a once daily insulin glargine (Lantus) dose of 25 units and metformin 500 mg twice daily. Blood sugars were rarely above 200. The patient was in excruciating pain and diagnosed with a rheumatoid arthritis flare requiring a burst of prednisone at 20 mg daily for 14 days and then scheduled to reevaluate the dose. While receiving this prednisone burst, blood sugars were above 300 at times, and the Lantus was titrated up. I've seen cases where blood sugars in the 400-500+ range are possible depending upon the dose of prednisone and other factors. It's really important to remember how short term changes in medications can really throw off good management of a condition. One other important thing to remember about cases like this is when that prednisone burst is over, blood sugars in most cases will return back to baseline. If medications were adjusted during this burst, the doses may now need to be readjusted following completion.

What to do With an A1C and the Rest of the Story

How should we interpret an A1C? For the experienced clinician, this is a very simple question, but I occasionally see orders for A1C's at a rate more frequently than every three months. Remember that an A1C is an average blood sugar over a period of approximately three months. This can vary a little bit, but thinking about this fact, what value would an A1C monthly provide?

If you ever see an order for a monthly A1C (or even more frequently than that), question it with boldness. I've seen a few recently where medication changes have been made and then two weeks or a month later an order is made for an A1C. I suspect in the majority of cases I've come across, it is an oversight by the primary provider. The only potential benefit you could get from checking it more frequently than every three months is to get an overall trend in the direction of the A1C. However, we can easily do this through blood sugar monitoring. Blood sugar checks are instantaneous and ideally should be varied throughout different times of the day to really get a full picture of how blood sugar fluctuates.

HbA1c (%)	eAG (mg/dl)
5	97
6	126
7	154
8	183
9	212
10	240
11	269
12	298

A1C to Average Blood Sugar Chart
Chart via Mayoclinic.org

Here's an example where A1C alone (without blood sugars) can be totally misleading. A 77 year old with type

2 diabetes currently taking glipizide 5 mg daily has an A1C of 6.4. Great A1C right? Great diabetes care right? At goal right? The number is good, but this is an average. This patient had blood sugars ranging from the 40's to 400's. When you see an A1C, remember that it contributes to the story, but it doesn't complete the story and sometimes may even be misleading.

That same patient could have blood sugars from 80-200 and be extremely well managed, but the A1C alone cannot give you that information.

Warfarin (Coumadin) and NSAIDs

The interaction between warfarin and NSAIDs (Advil, Aleve, Nabumetone, etc.) is probably one of the worst drug-drug interactions in the elderly; in fact, the AMDA (American Medical Directors Association) lists it as one of its top ten in long-term-care/geriatrics. NSAIDs can cause issues with GI bleeding and ulcers by themselves. The addition of an NSAID on top of warfarin can dramatically increase the risk of this bleeding. I've seen numerous cases of this, and we need to try to avoid using these drugs together if at all possible. If the healthcare team deems that this combination can't be avoided, then extra careful monitoring is of high importance.

Treating Dementia Related Behaviors

Treating dementia related behaviors is arguably one of the greatest challenges in the elderly. I nearly daily get asked questions about behaviors associated with dementia. Often these patients can be aggressive, hit, spit, kick, swear, hallucinate, be sexually inappropriate, or have delusions. I was once asked, "What is the best medication to treat these behaviors?" I relate that question to what is the best antibiotic to use. If there was one miracle medication that worked, every patient would be on it. It really depends upon what you are trying to treat, and often we can do an adequate job of treating these behaviors without medications. Identifying the root cause of the behavior is of highest importance.

There are many questions to ask when assessing new or abnormal behavioral symptoms. Here's just a few to focus on from the start:

1. Identify the specific behaviors, and be sure to relay this information to the clinicians/caregivers who are helping in making decisions.
2. When did these behaviors start and what time(s) of the day do they happen?
3. Can we correlate the start of new behaviors to anything else? (i.e. fall, medication, pain, stroke, family crisis, infection, change in environmental factors, etc.)

Constipation

Constipation is a massive topic especially in the elderly with many disease states and medications that can contribute. I frequently see patients on 2, 3, or 4 different laxatives at a time. Periodically, I do come across some duplication. I had a resident on oral bisacodyl (Dulcolax), a stimulant laxative, placed on Senna, another stimulant laxative. Both were at low doses, so it was a simple fix to discontinue one and titrate up on the other one. My best advice to minimize the use or to avoid potential overuse is to really dig into that med list. Many of the individuals that are on multiple laxatives are also on numerous medications that may contribute to constipation. Anticholinergics and opioids are the two classes of medications that come to my mind first when trying to identify meds that may be worsening constipation. We can't always get rid of these medications or even reduce them, but it's a good place to start before adding more medications.

Clinical Case Review

This is a very simple case, and I just wanted to highlight a few things that come to my attention as I'm reviewing this list. Obviously we can't tell diagnosis/subjective/objective info from a simple medication list, but it can help get you in the mindset of formulating questions and identifying clinical medication problems.

<u>Current Medications:</u>
Vitamin B12 1000 mcg IM q month
Aspirin 81 mg daily
Rivastigmine (Exelon) 3 mg twice daily
Tiotropium (Spiriva) 18 mcg – 1 cap by inhalation daily
Lisinopril 20 mg 1 tab daily
Levothyroxine (Synthroid) 75 mcg 1 tab daily

At first glance, lab monitoring is going to be important with the levothyroxine, lisinopril, B12, and maybe aspirin (especially if anemia history or symptoms of anemia). None of the doses seem abnormal, all pretty standard. Tiotropium is an inhaled anticholinergic, but it isn't absorbed systemically at a very high rate, so I clinically wouldn't worry very much about it potentially blocking the effects of the rivastigmine (for suspected dementia). Rivastigmine is at a moderate dose. I'd be interested to know if this patient tried a higher dose and didn't tolerate it or if their provider did not want to try to maximize the dose for another reason? With the tiotropium (usually used for COPD), it'd be nice to know their respiratory history to see if they ever experience acute symptoms that would require them to have a rescue inhaler.

Using Side Effects As Treatment

Excessive weight loss in the younger population tends to be less of a problem than weight gain (with a few exceptions like eating disorders). However, in the elderly, there are definitely situations where weight loss can be problematic. In these instances, we must rule out medications first as there are many medications that can cause weight loss in the elderly. The acetylcholinesterase inhibitors (donepezil, etc.) and digoxin are a couple examples of medications that need to be monitored for this potential adverse effect. There are obviously medical conditions that can cause weight loss as well. While keeping this in mind, there are times when we can't identify medications or a new diagnosis as the cause for a troublesome weight loss. Let's take into account that a patient may have a corresponding depression as well as insomnia. This is the type of case where we can try to kill two or three birds with one stone. Say we have a patient on an antidepressant and insomnia medication with a new problem of weight loss. I frequently see mirtazapine (Remeron) used in this case as it has a side effect profile that tends to cause weight gain and sedation as well as being indicated for the treatment of depression.

Fentanyl Patches Can Be Extremely Dangerous!

In my practice, I see frequent problems and questions on fentanyl (Duragesic) patches. I must highlight how potent fentanyl patches are! A 25 mcg/h patch has a ballpark equivalent to oral morphine of 60-134 mg daily per Lexicomp! A 50 mcg/h patch is approximately double that in oral equivalent of morphine per day. A 100 mcg/h patch oral morphine equivalent is in the ballpark of 315-404 mg per day. So if a patch is lost whether you are at home, an assisted living, nursing home, or other institution, you better take it seriously!

Tramadol (Ultram)

This medication is frequently used for various types of pain and is a controlled substance in the US. It definitely has opioid activity, so common side effects are the usual constipation, sedation, etc. and are similar to other opioids. One of the unique and unfortunate side effects of this medication is that it can lower seizure threshold. I've certainly seen cases where the patient had a seizure and was on this medication. How much of a role it played in a patient's seizure can be difficult to identify sometimes. If there are other analgesic options for patients that have a seizure history, why would you take that chance?

Pregabalin (Lyrica) Case

I often see orders for drugs two or three times daily, and while this can be necessary, sometimes it may not be. There can also be significant cost factors at play when using medications multiple times per day. Pregabalin is flat priced per Medi-span. What does this mean? It means that 1 capsule of 25 mg is the same cost as 1 capsule of 50 mg or 1 capsule of 75 mg and so on. I see pregabalin used most often for neuropathy symptoms. It has action similar to gabapentin (Neurontin). Pregabalin is priced at over $300/month for 90 capsules per Medi-span. I had a patient receiving 50 mg three times daily for neuropathy, and they were doing well with their pain management. Reducing the dose was not deemed appropriate. In this case, we were able to successfully transition the patient from 50 mg three times daily to 75 mg twice daily. There are many factors that can go into whether transitions like this are appropriate, but we should always be mindful of costs when medications could be changed without changing the quality of care. You could make the argument that care was actually improved at a lower cost because the patient had improved quality of life with less pill burden (less pills taken per day). Pharmacokinetics certainly matters in this case, and what you're treating certainly matters as well. This change allowed a savings of over a hundred dollars a month. If pregabalin was being used for seizures, we'd certainly be a little more cautious and maybe less likely to try a transition like this depending upon the situation.

"Treating" Behaviors in the Elderly

The topic of psych medications in general is very challenging to say the least; I believe it is much more of an art than science when compared to heart failure and other conditions with better set guidelines. The problem I run into frequently, especially in geriatrics, is where other contributing factors to new behaviors are not addressed or ruled out. Here's a great example of that: I had a resident placed on lorazepam (Ativan) as needed for anxiety and asked the nurse if it was working well and how often they needed it. Lorazepam is certainly not the greatest drug as far as adverse effects go, especially in the elderly. With all benzodiazepines (lorazepam, clonazepam, alprazolam, temazepam, etc.), if you remember effects similar to alcohol, you'll remember most of the side effects of the benzo's. Falls, confusion, and sedation certainly can happen and must be monitored for if lorazepam is initiated. The nurse informed me that since the resident started nicotine replacement products, she did not need the lorazepam. The patient was going through nicotine withdrawal symptoms and was having negative "behaviors" because of it. So here's a classic case where a patient received a medication to try to treat symptoms of something else that could've easily be resolved upon adequate investigation.

Discontinuing Medications in the Elderly

You're probably aware I'm an advocate for simple, rationale use of medications. This means that at times we might consider reducing or discontinuing medications that may not be appropriate anymore for various reasons. There is a right way to discontinue medications, and when you hear the geriatric mantra of "start low, go slow", the "go slow" applies to discontinuing or reducing medications as well as increasing medications (with a few exceptions).

Here's an example: A patient was on metoclopramide (Reglan) 10 mg four times daily for about 6-12 months for issues with nausea and vomiting. The patient was started at 5 mg twice daily and titrated upward over a period of a couple months to her current dosing. She did not have gastroparesis and did not have any GI symptoms for the last month or two. The physician had been questioned if this medication could possibly be reduced as the patient had been asymptomatic for a while. I've seen prescribers discontinue this dose before, and my simple question is why? In the absence of adverse effects or serious drug interactions, why pull out the rug without slowly tapering? The medication was tapered up slowly, so why increase the likelihood of failing off of the medication by going to all or none?

BCPS

If you're a pharmacist, you are probably noticing that board certification is on the rise and often a recommendation or requirement for many clinical pharmacy positions. Here are some of my thoughts on board certification and its importance.

My BCPS Exam Experience

BCPS stands for Board Certified Pharmacotherapy Specialist. I've put together a little summary of what my BCPS exam experience was like.

So my mind would not let me sleep, and felt I needed to do a little more cramming for my BCPS exam on the morning of the exam. At 4:30am I got myself ready and stopped by a local Perkins near the testing center to get my energy up and get those last few clinical pearls in my head before the 5 hour exam began.

The huge challenge of the exam is the variety and scope of the exam – basically anything and everything. There were definitely a few questions where I could've closed my eyes and picked one, but I felt as if I could at least narrow down the majority to at least two or three different choices which should help my odds of passing. I'm thankful it's over and am ready to accept whatever fate it brings.

There was one thing that really jumped out at me after the test was over…the survey. You're probably thinking what? Who cares about the survey after the exam? I felt the same way. I wanted to go take a nap. I didn't want to do it after racking my brain through 200 questions of random pharmacy topics and statistics. My conscience got the better of me, and I did it. Where am I going with this? I got nearly to the end and the question went something like "why did you take this exam", check all that apply. There were about 7 or 8 options, and I checked the first one which was career advancement and then started going down the list. Promotion, increased status, bonus, employer paid for it, and a couple others were on the list. There was one reason that did not appear in the list that I was really surprised that the creators of the survey didn't even list as a possibility. What about to improve the lives of my patients? This is not intended to float my own boat and I apologize if it sounds that way, but I know a couple pharmacists who wanted to take the exam to improve their skills and become better pharmacists so they are able to provide a higher quality of patient care. I'm not delusional and know that some of those other factors certainly play a role in deciding to take an exam like this, but to not have some sort of a statement about patient care was shocking. I'd be interested in knowing who creates the survey and if anyone proofs it. In defense of the survey, there was an "other" box but no line to write anything in. Good luck to anyone else who is taking the challenge this year! Just my two cents on the BCPS exam!

Does Credentialing Really Matter?

I had a doctor a year or two ago ask for my input on a patient that she was struggling with. Warfarin and INR management was the topic. I think I recall the term "roller coaster" when the physician described the case to me. So we sat and chatted for a few minutes and put our brains together as to what could cause this gentleman's INR to be all over the place. Diet changes, adherence, new medications, discontinued medications, over-the-counter use, disease state changes, different generics being dispensed, etc. Even the possibility of a medication error was considered. None of this made any sense to the physician as she felt the patient had always been very trustworthy. She had also asked him all those questions several times. I had asked if he was a candidate for one of the newer anticoagulants, but the physician did not feel he was. I was perplexed like she was on what to do with this patient. Where am I going with this?

I tell you this story because there's been a lot of chatter going on about the value of board certification for pharmacists. There are all sorts of specialties now: oncology, pediatrics, pharmacotherapy, geriatrics, and on and on... I've worked clinically for about 6 years since I graduated in 2009 and have worked closely with a lot of really good people, many of whom have worked 10+ years in the field as clinical pharmacists. Would I rather have board certification or the experiences I've had? The experience certainly trumps the certification. However, I tell you the above story because in the effort of preparing for the BCPS exam, I learned (or relearned) that patients with variable INR's can sometimes be prescribed supplemental vitamin K to help with difficult management*. This bit of information would've been nice to remember when discussing this case, allowing me to give the patient and doctor one more option.

The benefit of certification is not the letters or passing the test, the gold is found from the acquisition of information through time invested in preparing for the exam, which ultimately will help you do your job of helping patients better.

*Reference: Vitamin K supplementation to decrease variability of International Normalized Ratio in patients on vitamin K antagonists: a literature review
http://www.ncbi.nlm.nih.gov/pubmed/18695375

My One Minute BCPS Study Guide

A few folks out there have created a BCPS study guide that I was extremely grateful to have as I prepared to take and pass my exam. I wanted to give you my most important tips for passing the BCPS exam.

Tip 1: This has been stated by many pharmacists, but the key to passing this exam starts and ends with statistics. In creating my practice exam, I felt like I had way too many study design/biostatistics/regulatory questions, but just look at the percentage layout of the exam. BPS lists that percentage as 25% of the exam. That's 50 out of 200 questions! Don't be caught off guard.

Tip 2: Know your weaknesses. Any BCPS study guide should be individualized. In my case, I am not an expert ICU or HIV pharmacist. I hit those areas (along with statistics, did I get my point across in Tip 1!?) more than the rest. Geriatrics is my baby, so I didn't need to hammer that too hard.

Tip 3: Study. This is a simple one. Any good BCPS study guide will have a heavy focus on the study aspect. In all seriousness, if it has been a while since you've been in school or have taken another certification exam, I would suggest you start studying sooner rather than later. I believe that residents and younger graduates who did well in college will have an easier time getting into that groove. They also may have an easier time being current on topics that they don't use much in their practice versus the pharmacist that may not have intensely studied an HIV drug in 10-20 years.

Tip 4: Answer every question! This is right from BPS website "It is to the candidate's advantage to answer every question on the examination. There is no penalty in the scoring formula for guessing." You have to set a decent pace if you are a slow test taker and you have to answer every question! Practice questions will certainly help you better prepare and ease your fear when you take the real BCPS exam.

Tip 5: Odds are likely if you've been working clinically for a while, you will have a good grasp on basic lab values. If you don't know basic lab values, you will find yourself looking them up frequently which if you are a moderate to slow test taker, may cost you dearly (see Tip 4). I would suggest you memorize some basic ones if you haven't already – BMP, CBC, LFT, and some of the major narrow therapeutic index drugs like phenytoin, digoxin, lithium, etc.

Pharmacist Board Certification: Which one is Right for You?

There has been growing interest in pharmacist board certification. I think it will only be increasing as the job market seems to be tightening up. Another reason for the increase might be the steady progression toward provider status. I've been asked by several pharmacists; which one should I try to obtain?

There are a lot of board certifications now available for pharmacists: Pharmacotherapy, Ambulatory Care, Geriatrics, Oncology, Pediatrics, Psychiatry, etc. I can't tell you exactly which one is right for you, but I can tell you my thought process in deciding to become a Certified Geriatric Pharmacist (CGP) and Board Certified Pharmacotherapy Specialist (BCPS).

I took my CGP exam a few years back now and don't regret it. I work primarily in geriatrics, and the certification made a lot of sense given a significant amount of my work as a clinical pharmacist is done in long term care (heavily geriatrics).

Why did I do BCPS? I view BCPS as the most universal certification. The topics covered in this certification are extensive and include everything from pediatrics, critical care, geriatrics, ambulatory care, and so on. I want to fully disclose that I do have a 200 question BCPS mock exam for sale at meded101.com; however, I took the BCPS exam long before I ever considered creating a practice exam. For your reference, per accp.com, about 14,000 pharmacists have BCPS certification. About 1,500 have ambulatory care and oncology respectively, the next two most popular certifications from BPS (data reported from 2013).

Which pharmacist board certification is right for you? My take: If you know 100% you want to practice in a particular area/specialty of pharmacy for the rest of your career, doing a specific certification like oncology makes a lot of sense. If you are not exactly sure where your career path will take you as many younger pharmacists are not, I would probably recommend the BCPS certification.

BCPS Practice Exam and Study Guide

In addition to the premium 200 question BCPS mock exam and Biostatistics Study Guide, I put together a 10 Question Free BCPS Practice Exam that you should check out if interested in learning more about Board Certification. All of the above three BCPS tools can be found at meded101.com. For pharmacy students, I've also created

NAPLEX content (including a mock exam) to help prepare you for that examination.

MEDICATION MISTAKES

Warfarin (Coumadin) Dosing

Warfarin is a high risk medication. I have had the opportunity to frequently review medication errors at dozens of healthcare facilities. Coumadin is a tricky drug to dose and because of this, it can sometimes require odd dosing schedules. I've seen dosing all over the place. Someone may get 5 mg 2 days per week, and 2.5 mg the rest of the week or 5 mg one day a week, and 2.5 mg 6 days a week. Common sense tells us that the more complex and less routine the dosing regimen is, the more likely it is that an error will occur. It is challenging to always create a consistent daily dose, but it would certainly be ideal to do a standard daily dose to minimize risk of confusing orders.

Fentanyl Patches for Acute Pain

Fentanyl patches are easy to use…just slap it on right? I definitely see nurses ask for these patches fairly frequently. They are much easier for administration and less time consuming than oral dosage forms that may have to be given multiple times per day. There are many cases I've seen where fentanyl patches are NOT appropriate. One such case is in the event of acute pain. Per Lexicomp, fentanyl patches have an onset of 6 hours and may not begin to have full effect for at least 12 to 24 hours. In one case I came across, a resident was sent to the ER for a fall and prescribed a fentanyl patch with no prn pain med available. Would you like to be that patient and wait at least 6 hours before the analgesic effects even start? Clearly in pain, staff had to call back and get an order for a prn opioid to go with the fentanyl. One other important point I want to make on fentanyl patches; the frequency of changing the patch is a funky timeframe. They are usually changed every third day. I frequently see medication errors in which the patch got left on or didn't get changed appropriately. It's another one of those cases where there isn't a routine (i.e. daily), and it makes it easier to make an error.

Levothyroxine Medication Error

I had a case a while back where a patient had an elevated TSH at around 13. The patient was on a levothyroxine dose of 112 mcg 2 tablets daily. If you put yourself in the shoes of the provider, you can imagine seeing a large number of faxes/orders that you have to review in a day and this one slipping by. The provider got the fax and inadvertently wrote for 125 mcg daily, thinking he was increasing the dose. In reality, it was a significant decrease making the patient even more hypothyroid. A good reminder for dosing levothyroxine according to TSH is that it is counterintuitive. If TSH is high, the dose is usually increased. If the TSH is low, it indicates too much thyroid hormone, and the dose should be reduced. If you've worked in healthcare for a while, you have probably seen errors happen because of 1/2 tab orders or 2 tab orders. Another important point is always being on the lookout for abnormally large changes in dosing as this one slipped by the pharmacy and nursing audits. If there is any doubt in your mind about the order, be sure to confirm with the provider that wrote for the order. You can place the blame where you want to on this case, but it doesn't really matter as the end result is the same – the patient got the wrong dose.

Med Rec 101

Medication reconciliation (often called "med rec") can be pretty boring, but med rec done right can be lifesaving. An 89 year old male was hospitalized with a GI bleed and significant anemia. This patient's baseline hemoglobin was already in the 10-11 mg/dl range prior to the GI bleed secondary to chronic kidney disease. Upon discharge from the hospital, anemia was improving, but hemoglobin was still only around 8 mg/dl. It was obvious from reading the progress notes from the hospital stay that his aspirin was not going to be continued due to GI bleed risk. On the discharge medication reconciliation form, the aspirin was checked to be discontinued. What the staff didn't realize was that this form had changed, and when I checked the active medication list, this patient was still receiving the aspirin. This had slipped by two healthcare professionals because their med rec form had changed (i.e. they weren't used to identifying the medication orders on that new form). This patient did end up receiving the aspirin for a couple weeks, fortunately without issue. It is very easy to get into "auto-pilot" mode, but we must think critically at all times! Medication Reconciliation is another one of my top 30 medication mistakes (a free resource that can be found at meded101.com).

Memantine (Namenda) Conversion

Many patients and healthcare professionals may not realize that different formulations of a product can have very different pharmacokinetics. Why does pharmacokinetics matter? An 88 year old patient was receiving memantine 5 mg in the morning and 10 mg in the evening for dementia. The physician noted this and was going to transition him to the XR formulation. The physician noted the dose and converted him to 14 mg daily of the XR formulation, obviously looking for the closest match to the total 15 mg that the patient was taking already. Because of the pharmacokinetic properties of Namenda XR versus the regular release, this patient was under dosed on what he was previously receiving. No issues were noted on this incorrect transition, but potential was obviously there. When converting the same drug between different dosage forms, be sure to look up differences in pharmacokinetics to prevent under or overdosing the patient.

Life Threatening Morphine Errors

This is an incredibly important topic that I need to address. Math. I said it, please don't stop reading, this may help you or someone you care about prevent a devastating medication error. While most medication errors do not impact patient health, there is a medication error I see happen that can: errors involving concentrations of liquid dosage forms. Liquid oral morphine is a classic example of a drug that has numerous strengths and liquid concentrations. The concentrations I see most often are the concentrated morphine at 20mg/ml and occasionally 10mg/5ml. If these two concentrations get messed up, you are looking at a 10-fold error. Take 2.5 ml of the 10mg/5ml dose, and you get a 5 mg dose. If the concentrated morphine was (in error) dispensed, administered, or written for, you are looking at a 50 mg dose! If you get easily confused with these conversions, you must ask for help to double check your work. Please remember to look and think about the concentration of a liquid you are using as I've seen this situation end badly before and don't want to see it happen again.

1/2 Tabs, 2 Tabs, 3 Tabs = Medication Errors

Medication errors are always a challenging topic to address because it is no fun to make an error, and there is always the possibility of patient harm due to an error. Here's a case example where the way an order is written can make things more difficult to understand. A 68 year old nursing home resident was having some issues with pain and was prescribed acetaminophen (Tylenol) 500 mg 2 tablets twice daily. It may look pretty simple to interpret when it's typed out here, but factor in handwriting concerns, and it's easy to overlook the "2" in the order. Whenever I see orders with 2 tabs, 3 tabs, ½ tabs, etc., there's a little warning light bulb that goes off in my head, and it's because of experience. I've seen so many errors happen due to pharmacists, nurses, and doctors missing the "2" in this scenario. That's exactly what happened in this case. The order at the nursing home was transcribed as 500 mg twice daily. The patient outcome was insignificant (which is the case with the majority of medication errors) as the patient's pain was well managed on the lower dose. You could certainly imagine this potentially not turning out as well if this was a higher risk medication like a seizure medication, anticoagulant, or high dose opioid.

Knowing Brand Name Versus Generic Name

This is often a hot button issue with students. In the US, we work with medications that don't always have the same name. So what's more important, knowing the brand name or generic name? Let me give you an answer you probably won't like hearing. You need to know both.

Let's use warfarin as our example. The generic name is warfarin, but also has the brand name of Coumadin. Let's make it more confusing as some clinicians will use Jantoven, another brand name extension. To be honest, this is a stupid system. We are asking for patients to get hurt. Unfortunately, I can't prevent doctors, nurses, or other pharmacists from using any of these terms, so I have to know them all, and you need to as well. If you don't, you need to look them up.

I noted that an INR had not been drawn on a new resident to a LTC facility. I had left a note to the nurse to please take care of this today which led to a follow up phone call where the nurse had told me the resident was not on Coumadin (warfarin). Don't get me wrong, I've made mistakes, but remembered looking at this case two or three times. I ended up going back to the med list and the nurse was right, he was not on Coumadin, but he was on Jantoven, a less common brand name of warfarin. You might ask why the nurse didn't look it up which is a legitimate question, but when you see a medication list of 20+ medications, things are much more likely to get missed. If you don't know what a medication is, you have no clue how to safely monitor that medication. Look it up.

Pain and Capsaicin Products

I occasionally see capsaicin products (creams, gels, etc.) used for the treatment of pain. I also frequently see as needed orders for this medication. This medication applied topically is recommended to be used 3-4 times per day to affected area with best results occurring 2-4 weeks after continued use (per Lexicomp). This repeated application causes the depletion of substance P, a chemomediator involved in pain impulses. So clinically, what does this mean? This medication most likely will not work without consistent administration, so an as needed order as I've seen probably dozens of times will likely be ineffective. Time, effort, and money may potentially be wasted due to the drug not be utilized appropriately.

Potassium and ACE Inhibitors

The longer I live, the more I realize how important the simple things in life are. Communication, whether in your personal life or in your work, is so important. Here's a great example of a missed opportunity due to ineffective or inadequate communication. Labs were drawn on a patient that revealed an elevated potassium, so a fax was sent to the physician from a nursing home. The provider noted the potassium to be at 5.9 mEq/L (normal range 3.5-5.1 depending upon lab) and asked the question, "Are they on any potassium supplements?" The nurse responded with "no". The resident wasn't on a potassium supplement, but she was on an ACE Inhibitor (lisinopril, enalapril, ramipril, etc.), a very common cause of hyperkalemia. Had the nurse been a little stronger clinically or been able to pay a little closer attention to the med list, she could've been able to prevent possible unnecessary use of sodium polystyrene (Kayexalate). The physician should've had more time to look into the medication list as well, but we don't live in a perfect world all the time. Had the attending physician asked a different, more specific question, it might have prompted the nurse to look a little more closely as well.

Acetazolamide for Glaucoma

A 56 year old male has a history of CHF, diabetes, osteoarthritis, and glaucoma.

Current Medications:
Aspirin 81 mg daily
Losartan 50 mg daily
Metoprolol 12.5 mg twice daily
Metolazone 2.5 mg three times per week
Furosemide 80 mg daily
Acetaminophen 500-1000 mg three times daily as needed
Glipizide XL 5 mg daily
Latanoprost eye drops at night

This gentleman had an appointment with his optometrist to have a further assessment of his glaucoma. Upon return, he was prescribed oral acetazolamide for glaucoma at 250 mg by mouth twice daily. The potassium level a few months before the acetazolamide was started was 3.5 mEq/L. It was unclear whether the primary physician was aware of the eye doctor appointment or if he had been notified, but he did not recall or anticipate any relevant medication changes. The eye doctor did not order any follow up lab work when the acetazolamide was ordered for glaucoma.

Acetazolamide is a carbonic anhydrase inhibitor that has a diuretic effect. This medication being utilized by itself would likely have a much lower risk of causing electrolyte abnormalities, but when used in combination with other potent diuretics like furosemide and metolazone, the outcome was a little scary. Another factor here was that the potassium was at the low end of normal (3.5 mEq/L) at baseline. When the kidney function and electrolytes were finally rechecked over a month following initiation of acetazolamide, the potassium was dangerously low at 2.7 mEq/L. This is a classic case where poor interdisciplinary communication and inattentiveness on many accounts led to the negative outcome.

Morphine Dosing & Tolerance

I want to demonstrate that opioids really have no maximum as far as dosing goes. So what does this mean, and how is it relevant? Individuals can develop tolerance to opioids which means that over time, they may need increasing doses to receive the same effects. Because of this, you may see patients on extremely high doses that would certainly be lethal to opiate naïve individuals (i.e. those who aren't on chronic opioids). I had an example of this a while ago where a patient on hospice was on 300mg of long acting morphine three times per day, as well as an as needed immediate release dose of 120 mg! That's the highest dose of opioid I had seen in quite some time. If you ever have to prescribe, administer, review or dispense this dose, it should scare the crap out of you. I have seen wrong patient med errors happen, and this is a case where it would likely have a chance to be fatal if given to the wrong individual. With usual morphine starting doses in the ballpark of 5-15 mg orally, you can really see how this tolerance effect is demonstrated.

Fentanyl Patch Dose Titration and Potential Overdose

Fentanyl patches take a long time to ramp up, which also means that it takes a little while to get to a steady state concentration. What does this mean clinically? I've seen a case where the dose was increased too quickly, and the absorption/concentration was not allowed to get to a steady state before the dose was increased further. The patch was being increased every three days, and it is usually recommended every 5-7 days (or 2 patch changes if using every 72 hours). The patient ended up with too much opioid ("snowed", lethargic, increased confusion, etc.)

which brings me to one other important point with fentanyl…if there is an overdose situation, the drug is still deposited in the skin and will not stop absorbing once the patch is simply removed. It will take in the ballpark of a day for that drug to get through the skin and half of it to be eliminated.

Phenytoin (Dilantin) Toxicity

I showed up to a long term care facility mid-afternoon and just caught the charge nurse as she was heading out early for the day. She asked me to take a look at a specific resident's medications as she felt that her condition was declining and they were wondering if she could do without some. This is always a red flag in my mind to rule out potential drug causes that could be attributed to the decline in condition. I probably wouldn't be writing this case if it wasn't drug related. The only order over the previous month was an increase in phenytoin from 300 mg per day to 600 mg per day. For most drugs you might think this isn't a big deal, but phenytoin isn't like most drugs as it has some abnormal kinetics (how the body affects drugs). Why this increase in maintenance dosing is problematic is because small increases in dose can lead to large changes in the blood concentration. This is a prime example why kinetics matters clinically as there are many situations where it is reasonable to simply double the dose. The resident had increasing lethargy, confusion, nausea and vomiting. Fortunately, the resident had been refusing some of the doses, so I estimated that she was receiving about 450 mg per day on average. The phenytoin level was checked and was in the toxic range at around 35 mcg/ml (normal range is 10-20). Hospitalization was avoided, and the resident returned to baseline once the drug was reduced.

Have a Healthy Respect for Long Acting Injectable Antipsychotics

An 81 year old female had a history of dementia related behaviors. Whenever you hear dementia related behaviors, do not jump to conclusions. Define the behaviors first. This particular patient refused medications, refused cares, was really nasty verbally to other residents, and would occasionally become aggressive with staff including trying to hit, pinch and bite.

This patient had multiple trials on various antidepressants and antianxiety medications which often happens in cases such as this. Nothing was working. Risperidone 0.25 mg twice daily was started and increased to 0.5 mg twice daily within a few weeks due to no improvement.

Nursing staff was getting incredibly frustrated with this patient and was seeking alternative solutions to manage the behaviors since the risperidone was not working and was also being refused multiple times. One of the nurses had remembered that long-acting haloperidol (Haldol) decanoate had worked really well on a resident they had in the past. The prescriber wrote for haloperidol decanoate 100 mg every 28 days.

First off, these long acting antipsychotics are extremely scary and should be used with the utmost respect. Think about giving a drug for 28+ days; you essentially can't take it back. If they have an allergy or intolerance, good luck. That's why test oral doses are typically given which can be a challenge if the patient is refusing medications.

Conversion from risperidone to haloperidol is not an exact science, but I assure you the dose of haloperidol decanoate prescribed was way too high! This is a SCARY WAY

TOO HIGH DOSE, especially in an 81 year old on a low dose of risperidone that she is frequently refusing anyway.

Long acting injectable antipsychotics are serious business. You have to make sure that other options have been exhausted first (especially in the elderly) and that you have a significant comfort level in how these medications are managed. Remember, once given, you can't take it back.

Inappropriate use of Fentanyl Patches

A 76 year old male recently had a hip fracture that required surgery. He was in a substantial amount of pain. Upon discharge from the hospital, he was admitted to a long term care facility for rehab. Acute pain management was the highest on the priority list, and the provider started a fentanyl patch 25 mcg as needed every three days. You could imagine my surprise when I saw this order. So what's wrong with a fentanyl patch as needed? Two major points:

1. Fentanyl patches are not meant for acute pain to begin with; they are meant for chronic pain.
2. Even more importantly, here's a prime example why knowing and learning pharmacokinetics matters. The onset of a fentanyl patch takes at least about 6 hours (per Lexicomp) to start having an effect which flies in the face of the premise of an as needed medication. As needed medications are meant to help treat a condition quickly. Would you want your patient in pain for at least 6 hours (probably much longer) before he started feeling any relief at all? The patient did request to use it as it was meant for his pain control, and not surprisingly, he did not get any acute pain relief from the patch. A substantial waste of money and time as well as not helping the patient!

PATIENT EXPERIENCE

Why Don't Younger People Get Vaccinated?

Vaccination is a controversial topic in the minds of some, and people have seriously strong opinions about this issue, so I approach it with that in mind. I personally see the impact of influenza outbreaks in nursing homes; it can be absolutely devastating in frail, elderly individuals. I also review that these residents get vaccinated and anecdotally, I can't say I see many side effects or bad outcomes from vaccination. I can't recall anyone ever getting hospitalized due to the vaccine. In my mind, the potential benefits of vaccination greatly outweigh the risks. Mild side effects do happen from time to time, but rarely is this ever a significant issue. If you are a young-middle aged adult in good health, you are probably going to survive if you get influenza without being vaccinated, but I ask you to think about the ones around you who may not be in as good of health. I spoke with a doctor who was very frustrated with the vaccination rate in younger individuals, and she made a great point about that. She said that concerns over vaccines in older individuals are much less when compared to the horrible diseases that they have seen prevented. Younger individuals don't have experience with how severe some of the diseases that vaccines now prevent really are. I'm sure there are cases of severe reactions out there, and I fully respect not getting vaccinated because of that reason. Maybe the most persuasive argument I can make is what I do with my children, and all I can say to you is that they get vaccinated.

Should You Only Use One Pharmacy?

I saw an article posted on KevinMD.com that was written last year or so; it prompted me to look at other articles similar to this. I feel this article really gives a telling insight into the way many (non-pharmacy) medical professionals feel about pharmacists who dispense medications. In the article, a medical student describes the situation where warfarin is 15 dollars at one pharmacy and 4 dollars at another. The article goes on to discuss the wide differences in the cost of drugs at different pharmacies. For those not in the world of pharmacy, I'm sure it's an interesting read and leads the reader to believe that there is no value in getting your prescriptions at the same pharmacy. I am all for transparency and competition, but I'm going to save that discussion for another day. I believe this article really gives you the sense that dispensing pharmacists provide zero value other than the product they dispense, but I guess that's the problem when you have been historically attached to the sale of a product. I'm not intending to tear down this writer who wrote the article, but I am asking healthcare professionals and pharmacists to look inward and a little deeper at what a pharmacist can and does provide. I believe there is a significant proportion of healthcare providers (non-pharmacy) who feel as if dispensing pharmacists are simply making sure the correct drug and quantity are in the bottle. For example, the author of this article compared buying a pack of gum to getting your prescription filled. For cash paying patients, when your sole focus is cost, it's a no brain decision...go buy the Coumadin, Lasix, or Zithromax at the cheapest location. However, let's dig a little deeper than that. Let's say Coumadin is cheaper at pharmacy A. Go get your Coumadin there. Now, that same patient gets put on Bactrim – pharmacy B sells this drug at a much cheaper price than pharmacy A. Would pharmacy B know that the patient is on Coumadin and that there is potential for a significant drug interaction? Obviously any computer program designed to help aid in identifying interactions is useless in this case. The pharmacist might know that the patient is on Coumadin, or identify that upon adequate questioning, but I can guarantee you that it is not nearly as likely if the patient received all his or her prescriptions at one pharmacy. I've seen people get hospitalized due to this interaction. Working in healthcare, I understand that nurses, pharmacists including myself, and doctors all make mistakes. A pharmacist is a critical final check before the drug reaches the patient to help prevent hospitalizations, injuries, and deaths. There is definitely a long way to go in educating the public as well as other healthcare professionals as to what pharmacists know and can do. So is the 15 dollar Coumadin actually cheaper than 4 dollar Coumadin? I will let you decide.

Patient Experience with Insulin Pens

I can remember doing a home visit with a patient who had recently been discharged from the hospital. This particular individual had a recent CHF exacerbation as well as pneumonia. I will never forget the experience that made me reflect upon how I try to educate patients. We had been discussing all of his medications, going through them one by one, making sure doses were correct, and he knew what to look out for with the recent changes to his medication regimen. I've always tried to ask patients at least two or three different times if they have any questions. Some may get annoyed, but I'd rather risk that than not having an important question asked. When we were wrapping up, I asked him one last time if he had any questions. "Yeah, you know what, I do need to ask you a question," he stated as he was getting up out of his chair. He went to the kitchen and came back with an insulin pen, tossed it to me, and said, "What do I do with this?" It would've been interesting to see the look on my face as I had no idea what he meant as we had gone through his insulin regimen already, and he had been using insulin for years. "They sent this home with me from the hospital, and I don't know how to use it," he stated. Puzzled, I informed him that this is insulin. He then went and retrieved his vial of insulin from the fridge. In what I anticipated was an effort not to waste the insulin pen, he had received an insulin pen upon hospital discharge that he had no idea how to use. He also had no needles for the pen. It's vitally important to ask questions, and obviously an important question about whether the patient knew how to use an insulin pen was not asked at the hospital. This situation ended without issue, but the potential was there for the patient to get into some real trouble.

Insurance Company Causes Negative Patient Outcome

Many patients get medication management suggestions from their insurance companies addressed to their primary physician. A patient who had diabetes and CHF was not on an ACE Inhibitor or an ARB which are commonly recommended as standard of care for hypertension and these coexisting conditions. In following this patient, there were records that an ACE inhibitor had been tried in the past and had been discontinued due to hyperkalemia (elevated potassium). The patient had recently switched to a new physician who received the letter and proceeded to put this patient on lisinopril. Sure enough, after checking some lab work, the lisinopril caused hyperkalemia again and was discontinued. A few questions I'd like you to think about:

1. Should the new provider have caught this and is he totally responsible?

2. Should the adverse effect have been noted in the allergy/intolerance list? Many adverse effects in my experience are not added to this list.

3. Did the insurance company letter set the patient/prescriber up for this negative outcome, and should insurances send out these letters?

Discontinuing Lab Work With Medications

While reviewing a patient's medications and pertinent medical history, I occasionally will come across a lab that was drawn on an individual that is totally puzzling to me. You may see Coumadin discontinued due to various reasons, but many times it is due to high risk of bleeding or something similar to this. What you need to remember to try to prevent unnecessary lab work is to discontinue associated lab monitoring with that medication (in this case, obviously INR). Other examples include discontinuing seizure medications (i.e.: Depakote) or statins in the setting of comfort or hospice type care. If you ever see medications that require routine lab work get discontinued, get the associated lab order discontinued BEFORE the lab is drawn unnecessarily. Save everyone some time, a potential needle stick, and money!

You Have Dementia – What is it like?

Who doesn't love a good game of Bingo? Someone came and asked me if I wanted to play the other day, and I thought it sounded like fun. The gentleman that invited me to play also said there would be prizes for the winners. What could be better than Bingo and prizes?!?!

I went and picked out a card from the stack and the game quickly started after that. Number after number was called, and I was getting closer to winning money! Finally B2 was called, "BINGO" I yelled. No one seemed to care, and everyone kept playing as if I had said nothing. I know how to play BINGO, and I've got a BINGO, why don't these people understand that? So I shut my mouth and kept playing, maybe if I get another BINGO, they will understand. I28 was called and again I had another BINGO, so I yelled it again, no response. What was going on? Someone told me that's not how you play this game. I didn't even know how to respond, so I waited one more time. Finally G53 was called, certainly someone will hear and listen to me now, I've got three BINGO's on my card – "BINGO" I yelled again. This time everyone playing wasn't just ignoring me; somehow I made them all mad. One actually said, "Get him out of here." I've played this game a million times and no one understands and is actually mad at me for saying that I have a bingo?

Put your empathy shoes on and start walking; this is what happens when someone with dementia tries to play a simple game of Blackout Bingo.

Transitions of Care – What Would You Think if You Just Escaped Death?

Transitions of care are an extremely vulnerable time for patients. Patients can be easily overwhelmed due to different medications, new diagnoses, new location, new people, and multiple things to learn. As healthcare professionals, it is easy to get into our work groove and forget to put ourselves in the shoes of our patients.

Hospitalization is one of the most stressful situations a patient can go through. Imagine that you have chest pain, get admitted to the hospital, and are newly diagnosed with a myocardial infarction (heart attack). If you make it through this situation and get discharged home, how would you feel, and what would your priorities be?

I think when we are educating these patients, we forget an important aspect. They are people; they have lives, families, and commitments just like the rest of us. If you nearly died, are in pain, and can't sleep well at night, would your focus be on whether you need to take metoprolol once or twice daily when you get home? What about taking your statin at night, would that be important to you? Or would you be thinking, how much longer do I have to live? How many times am I going to get to see my grandkids again? Or, will I get to go on that trip I've always wanted to do?

Even when caregivers are involved, they will have many of those same fears about their loved ones. Their focus is on their life, not their medications. Remember that.

I'm a huge advocate for close follow up of patients after they get home and start to get back to their usual routine. I think if you put yourself in the shoes of your patients, you'll realize what their priorities are going to be.

What Medications Are You On? No, Seriously.

You can know everything there is to know about medication management and still do the wrong thing for your patient. How is that possible?

Patients sometimes don't think that medications are actually medications. When we ask patients, "What medications are you currently taking," we think we are getting the correct answer including herbals, over-the-counters, and prescription medications. In my experience, this is seldom the case, and the real ugly part is, those medications can be a huge piece of the puzzle.

RS is a 79 year old female who is currently "taking"
Aspirin 325 mg daily
Hydroxyzine 50 mg at night for sleep
Torsemide 20 mg daily
Lisinopril 10 mg daily
Acetaminophen 1-2 tabs as needed, nearly nightly for pain

After we completed going through the medication list, a simple, quick review of systems was assessed. In this brief assessment, two more medications were uncovered as well as a complaint that she forgot to mention: Senna that she takes 2-3 tablets every day, Artificial Tears, as well as complaints of dry mouth. Pretty important pieces of the puzzle huh? Hydroxyzine is likely causing or contributing to these symptoms with its anticholinergic activity.

In this case, the patient did not feel that these were important enough to mention, but when used in the context of the other medications, the reporting of these medications is highly valuable to identify potential side effects. Always assume patients are taking more medications than what they report; more often than not, you'll be right.

Improper Phenytoin (Dilantin) Administration Leads to Seizure

A 78 year old patient on phenytoin suspension had a seizure, so a total phenytoin level was checked. (A free level probably would've been ideal in the case.) The level came back at around 4 mcg/ml which was unusual for this patient; his normal total level was in the 12-14 range. All factors were being considered as the potential cause in this change in concentration – drug interactions, were they taking the phenytoin, medication error, etc. A level was checked at 2 weeks, 4 weeks, and 6 weeks to try to help determine what was going on.

The levels came back at 18, 5, and 14 mcg/ml, respectively at each interval. No signs of toxicity were noted, but the large variation in the levels was troubling given that this patient had a seizure with a level around 4 mcg/ml.

After careful consultation with this patient, it was identified that she was simply not shaking the suspension. What ends up happening in this case is the medication settles to the bottom. When the bottle is full and not shaken, the medication is at the bottom, and the patient will not get an adequate dose. When the bottle is nearly empty, the patient will get a much more concentrated dose, and in this case explains the variation in the phenytoin levels perfectly. It's amazing how something so simple can be so critical and confusing in patient care.

Improper Steroid Administration Leads to Recurrent Thrush

A 63 year old female has a history of severe COPD. She is a smoker and is currently taking the following medications: ipratropium/albuterol as needed, budesonide and formoterol (Symbicort) 160/4.5 two inhalations twice daily, and tiotropium (Spiriva) inhalation once daily. Respiratory symptoms are fairly well managed.

She presents to the clinic with poor appetite, cough, and throat pain; she also complains of a gagging type feeling. Upon assessment, she's diagnosed with thrush and prescribed nystatin to treat the infection. The infection totally resolves within a couple of weeks.

Fast forward a couple months later, and the patient again presents with similar symptoms of irritated mouth and throat with difficulty swallowing. She is again diagnosed with a candida infection and treated with nystatin for 2-4 weeks with consideration of a longer time period depending upon response.

So, what was missed initially in this case? Upon investigation and careful questioning of the patient, it was discovered that she either was not educated or did not remember to rinse her mouth following administration of inhaled corticosteroids (which Symbicort contains). This is a classic example of why patient education is so important as well as identifies that new symptoms or medical problems could be caused or worsened by medications! In this case, the thrush could've possibly been prevented, saving our patient some pain and suffering.

Big Pharma Pulls a Fast One on Dementia Patients – Namenda XR

A few months back, I watched as many of the dementia patients I work with were transitioned from memantine (Namenda) to Namenda XR. Why? The company that makes Namenda was planning on stopping production. Why? The only logical conclusion I could come to is they must have needed the money.

The makers of both Namenda XR and Namenda will contend that Namenda XR is a superior product. If that's really true, why stop producing the regular Namenda? It should be obvious to healthcare professionals that Namenda XR is superior, and they shouldn't have anything to worry about, right? Obviously, they don't really believe that as they were trying to transition all patients off of Namenda to the XR formulation. The original Namenda will be going generic within the next year which will obviously be a substantial loss to the company. Is it right? Of course not. Is it legal? We will find out as there are lawsuits in the works.

To put some icing on this poorly tasting cake, there have been production problems with the XR formulation. So now some of those patients that I've seen switched to the XR have to be switched back to the original formulation they were on just a couple months before. Dementia patients and their caregivers have enough to worry about.

This may surprise you, but I'm all for Big Pharma. We need creativity. We need options to help provide the best possible care. We don't need stunts.

POLYPHARMACY

Students tend to really enjoy the polypharmacy medication reviews that you will find later in this section. I think the value in these mini cases is learning how you would prioritize the clinical thought process. The goal is to develop your thought process, not get "the answer" correct. If you change one variable from patient to patient, it can dramatically change the recommendation or medication adjustment you would make. Focus on developing your thought process and the questions you'd like to investigate, not the answer. No two patients are ever identical.

The 10 Commandments of Polypharmacy

I work with patients, nurses, doctors, pharmacists and other healthcare professionals every day who struggle with medication management. One of the biggest problems I run into is polypharmacy. Ten, twenty, even 30+ medications is something I come across on a daily basis. Here are my top ten ways that healthcare professionals can help minimize polypharmacy.

1. Thou shalt not start, ask for, dispense, or administer a medication without reviewing a medication list that is accurate, up to date, and complete with over-the counter medications and supplements
2. Thou shalt consider utilizing non-drug approaches and interventions to solve patient problems before initiating medication
3. Thou shalt assess if a medication is effective before adding a new medication for the same condition
4. Thou shalt consider any new symptom is an adverse effect of another medication until proved otherwise

5. Thou shalt not start a medication without an appropriate indication and assessing appropriate lab work

6. Thou shalt identify limits for medications not intended for chronic use as well as not continue a medication indefinitely for symptoms that have an expected short duration

7. Thou shalt not start a medication from a similar medication class without appropriate rationale

8. Thou shalt not initiate a medication without considering medications that may treat duplicate conditions – Kill two birds with one stone

9. Thou shalt consider eliminating or reducing medications at every medication review

10. Thou shalt be willing to accept risk in discontinuing a medication if they were willing to accept the risk of initiating a medication

After a C. Diff. Infection

A 78 year old male living in a long term care facility was recently prescribed a couple of different courses of antibiotics to treat recurrent respiratory infections. Treatment was eventually successful, but a few days following the final treatment with antibiotics, diarrhea started to develop. It started out fairly mild but was progressing to several loose stools per day. The physician was notified of the diarrhea, and nurses had wondered if loperamide (Imodium) would help resolve the issues. Loperamide 2 mg twice daily was prescribed, with additional doses after each loose stool as needed (up to a max of 16 mg/day). Even with loperamide, the loose stools did not completely resolve. Clostridium difficile testing was performed and it was indeed positive. The resident was treated with metronidazole which was successful. Diarrhea was 100% resolved, and the resident was without any lingering symptoms. In the effort and justified concern with treating the C. Diff. infection, what was forgotten about was that the resident was still on the loperamide months after the C. Diff. had been treated. The lesson here is to remember to avoid long term medication use for an obvious short term problem.

Drug Induced Nausea – The Clinical Thought Process

Stomach problems can often be a common issue in the elderly, and drug induced nausea can sometimes be a challenge to identify due to polypharmacy. If you look under adverse effects of medications, nausea is a side effect for virtually every medication. Here's a medication list to review for drug induced nausea.

<u>Current Medications:</u>
Aspirin 81 mg daily
Metformin 1000 mg twice daily
Duloxetine 30 mg daily
Omeprazole 20 mg daily
Acetaminophen 1,000 mg three times daily
Oxycodone/Acetaminophen 5/325 mg four times daily as needed
Donepezil 10 mg daily
Ondansetron 4 mg three times daily as needed

Focusing on the medications, the first critical question you should ask to identify possible causes of drug induced nausea is: When did it start? This is always one of the first questions I think of when assessing a case. Timing is so critical, not every time, but most of the time. Other questions might be: Are there other symptoms associated like loose stools, heartburn, weight loss, or other GI problems? What dose of each medication are they on (i.e. is it a high dose for that med)? Do they have a diagnosis that might cause their nausea? Is diet a contributing factor? Do they have bad times of the day or is it more constant? Just looking at the meds, from my experience, metformin and donepezil are the most probable to cause the issue. So, identifying if either of these has been recently started OR increased would be important considerations. Oxycodone/acetaminophen is also another possibility (need to watch out for acetaminophen limit as well). I'd like to know how much/if this patient is taking that and try to correlate that with the nausea as well.

Polypharmacy – What Does it Look Like?

I came across this medication list, and just wanted to give you a brief idea of some of the thoughts that go through a clinical pharmacist's head. Scary I know, but just stay with me, as you will most likely see something at the end of this case that you've never seen before. This is a real med list. I've spoken with a couple people who've been in the business a long time, and they can't recall a medication list quite like this either.

Current Medications:
Albuterol nebs four times daily
Alendronate 70 mg on Wednesdays
Artificial Tears one drop three times daily OU
Vitamin C 500 mg daily
Budesonide/Formoterol (Symbicort) 160/4.5, two puffs inhaled twice daily
Calcium with Vitamin D 500 mg daily
Cyanocobalamin 1,000 mcg IM monthly
Donepezil 5 mg at bedtime
Escitalopram 20 mg daily

Exemestane 25 mg daily for history of breast cancer
Fentanyl patch 50 mcg q72hr
Fluticasone 0.05% 2 sprays to each nostril daily
Gabapentin 600 mg three times daily
Glucosamine chondroitin 500 mg daily
Guaifenesin 600 mg twice daily
Levothyroxine 0.075 mg daily
Loratadine 10 mg daily
Meloxicam 15 mg daily
Morphine Sulfate ER 45 mg three times daily
Oxygen at 2 liters via nasal cannula

Certainly you need more information than a medication list to determine appropriateness of each medication that a patient is on. However, you can begin to form ideas in what you might change about a patient's medications, identify potential problems, and get your mindset geared as to what to try to look for when reviewing a medication list.

In going through this medication list, I look at a few respiratory medications and oxygen, obviously this is a patient with some serious respiratory issues, so we need to be mindful of that. All the doses look low to moderate with the exception of the opioids and gabapentin which is at a moderate dose. I would make sure to keep an eye out for side effects of gabapentin as well as kidney function. Gabapentin is eliminated through the kidney. This patient is certainly getting a significant amount of opioid with no noted constipation medication(s), so we need to monitor for that. She obviously has some serious pain management issues and ideally it would be nice to convert her from 2 long acting opioids (fentanyl and morphine ER) to one at some point in time. This patient doesn't have a prn opioid for breakthrough pain either...kind of bizarre for someone on that high of a dose of opioids. Donepezil could potentially be increased to maximize the potential benefit depending upon GI status and if it hasn't been tried in the past. She obviously has some sinus and/or allergy issues on guaifenesin, loratadine, and fluticasone – maybe we could try to wean those down at some point if symptoms are well controlled.

Some other thoughts to try to minimize this patient's medication load would be to look at vitamin C and what that is being used for, as well as the glucosamine. There may not be much pain benefit if using for osteoarthritis due to the large amount of opioids and the meloxicam. She is also on an NSAID (meloxicam), so we will need to do some lab monitoring there as well. A TSH needs to be monitored on levothyroxine. Those are just some of the ideas that went through my head by simply looking at the medication list without yet looking into symptoms/assessment/H&P/vitals, etc. There really wasn't anything too crazy about this case that I hadn't seen before. If you are a patient, you are probably thinking that this is a ton of medications. If you are in healthcare and work in geriatrics, this is probably nothing you haven't seen before. I deal with these lists on a daily basis. Helping physicians and nurses identify medication related problems is what I do, and from the above, you can get a small glimpse of that. What separated this case from others I've seen is that I flipped to the next page in the H&P and saw this:

Patanol twice daily to both eyes
Omeprazole 20 mg daily
Oxybutynin 5 mg twice daily
MiraLax 17 grams daily
Senokot 2 tablets twice daily
Carafate 1 gram by mouth four times daily
Timolol maleate 1 drop 0.5% twice daily
Trazodone 25 mg at bedtime
Tylenol 650 mg three times daily prn

Albuterol nebs 2.5 mg q4h prn
Artificial Tears 1 drop q4h prn
Tessalon Perles 100 mg q2h prn cough
Cepacol lozenges 1 lozenge by mouth prn q2h
Cyclobenzaprine 10 mg three times daily pm
Voltaren Gel 2 grams 1% gel topically qid prn to shoulders as needed
Colace 200 mg twice daily prn constipation
Lasix 20 mg daily prn every other day for edema
Mucinex 600 mg twice daily prn
Robitussin 5 mL q4h prn
Lactulose 5 mL orally daily prn constipation
Imodium prn diarrhea
Ativan 0.5 mg three times daily prn anxiety
Maalox 30 mL three times daily prn gastric distress
Milk of Magnesia 30 mL at bedtime prn constipation
Potassium chloride 40 mEq twice daily when prn Lasix dose is given
Sumatriptan succinate 50 mg four times daily prn migraines
Trazodone 50 mg at bedtime prn insomnia
Cortisporin 1 gram 1% topical three times daily as needed
Ben-Gay 1gram topically three times daily prn
Nystatin cream 30 grams topically twice daily prn
Vancomycin 1 gram IV daily
Rifampin 300 mg twice daily, for 10 days

Over 50 medications total! I was speechless, and pray that I will never see a medication list like this again!

Diagnosis: Polypharmacy

I can't help but smile when providers dictate that a patient has a diagnosis of polypharmacy. Let's cure that condition! These case studies are kind of challenging because you could go a few different directions, but they do certainly provide some educational opportunities!

Current Medications:
Diltiazem CD 120 mg daily
Aspirin 81 mg daily
Atorvastatin 40 mg daily
Lisinopril 10 mg daily
Insulin aspart (Novolog) 4 units three times daily with meals
Insulin glargine (Lantus) 25 units at bedtime
Metformin XR 2000 mg daily
Citalopram 20 mg daily
Lorazepam 0.5 mg as needed
Trazodone 100 mg at bedtime
Paroxetine 40 mg daily
Omeprazole 20 mg daily
Ondansetron 4 mg three times daily as needed
Tums as needed
Nitrofurantoin 100 mg daily
Ibuprofen 400 mg four times daily as needed
Gabapentin 400 mg three times daily
Meloxicam 15 mg daily
Budesonide 0.5 mg nebs twice daily
Albuterol nebs four times daily as needed

The big questions I would want to know first from the medication list:

1. I would like to know GI status with duplicate NSAIDs contributing to any symptoms – i.e. how often using ondansetron, Tums, etc. Also, metformin and the antibiotic could contribute if the patient is having GI complaints.
2. Obvious duplicate SSRI's (citalopram, paroxetine) – there better be a really good reason for that, although from my experience it's almost always a mistake. This patient

most likely does have some significant behavioral/psych concerns given the number of psych meds. Potentially neuropathy with gabapentin and maybe an SNRI would be something to consider. One other possible reason for two SSRI's could be a cross taper onto one from the other.

3. Kidney function is going to be very important as many drugs can affect or be affected by renal function (nitrofurantoin, metformin, NSAIDs, lisinopril).

4. Diabetes, HTN, Respiratory and Pain assessment are of course necessary based on this med list, but I'm trying to help you learn how to prioritize!

Amlodipine Simvastatin Interaction

Current Medications:
Alendronate 70 mg weekly
Norvasc 5 mg daily
Amlodipine 5 mg daily
Cephalexin 1 gram prior to dental appointments
Folic acid 1 mg tablet twice a day
Furosemide 20 mg daily
Gabapentin 300 mg twice a day
Insulin lispro 5 units before meals
Lansoprazole 30 mg daily
Insulin glargine 10 units twice a day
Losartan 100 mg daily
Methotrexate 25 mg injection weekly
Metoprolol 100 mg daily
Oxycodone CR 10 mg three times a day
Pramipexole 0.25 mg at bedtime
Sertraline 100 mg daily
Simvastatin 80 mg tablet, one-half tablet daily
Sumatriptan 50 mg tablet, one to two tablets for migraines
Solifenacin 5 mg daily

The interaction between amlodipine and simvastatin was the first thing I noticed. Currently, FDA recommends a max dose of simvastatin 20 mg daily if on amlodipine. Also, I noted that amlodipine is listed twice which is the generic name of Norvasc.

I can't help but wonder why they are using the methotrexate injection over tablets in this case, and along with that, what the indication is that it is being used for? Also, remember that folic acid supplementation is recommended with methotrexate which this patient is on. I would be interested to know why she is on a higher than usual daily dose of folic acid (2 mg instead of 1 mg).

A few other points that I would look into: Do they need a PRN analgesic for breakthrough pain? With alendronate use, I would look into why we aren't supplementing with vitamin D/calcium. This patient is getting 5 injections, and it would be nice to get that number down if possible (6 with methotrexate weekly). She is on a relatively low dose of Lantus that could maybe go to one injection depending upon history. The frequency of triptan use for migraine would be important to assess. Both gabapentin and amlodipine can contribute to edema issues, so I would look into furosemide timing/relationship. There are plenty of labs to be monitoring as well!

Diabetes Med List Review

Current Medications:
Aspirin EC 325 mg oral twice daily for one month
Vitamin C 500 mg oral daily at bedtime
Calcium 600 mg oral daily at bedtime
Vitamin D 2000 units oral daily at bedtime
Senokot S 1 tab oral daily

Clotrimazole 1% apply thin layer to affected area twice daily
Glipizide 20 mg daily and 10 mg daily at 1800 hours
Levothyroxine 75 mcg oral daily
Lisinopril 10 mg oral daily
Oxybutynin 1 patch weekly (replace old patch on weekends)
Pioglitazone 30 mg oral daily and 15 mg oral daily at bedtime
Simvastatin 20 mg oral daily at bedtime
Tramadol 50 mg oral q.6h. for pain
Dulcolax 10 mg rectal as needed
Glucose 15 grams oral every 15 minutes as needed for mild hypoglycemia
Glucagon 1 mg intramuscular q.15 minutes as needed for glucose less than 50 mg patient unconscious/not alert. May repeat once in 15 – 30 minutes if patient does not respond. Roll patient on her side to prevent aspiration. Notify MD when initiating for hypoglycemia
Milk of magnesia 30 mL oral at bedtime as needed
Oxycodone 5-15 mg every 3 hours as needed

Pretty extensive med list, and I'm going to pick out three points that need to be investigated. It's really hard to limit it to three, but that gives you all an opportunity to identify other potential problems!

She has orders for management of hypoglycemia here, she is on a very steep dose of glipizide. Even with limited information, it's pretty obvious to me that we need to monitor blood sugars very closely! She is on pioglitazone as well which is split up into two doses. This medication is usually given once daily, so I would need to investigate that further as well.

Oxybutynin patch is usually dosed twice weekly. That would certainly need to be addressed and make sure that it is correct, beneficial, and tolerable for the patient.

This appears to be a probable rehab patient with the aspirin dosed twice daily for one month. One thing I've come across several times is to make sure that anticoagulation/antiplatelet therapy gets addressed long term versus short term. In this case, there is no noted order to continue aspirin for CV prophylaxis, she is likely a candidate long term being on the statin with diabetes meds. GI and bleeding risk history certainly need to be assessed as well before continuing long term antiplatelet therapy.

If It's Not Broke, Don't Fix It – Defining Polypharmacy

I received this comment on meded101.com on the above diabetes med list review I posted: "While the comment on the dosing schedule for Actos and Oxybutynin are valid, we need keep in mind that manufacturers recommended dosing schedules are not a bible and we are treating people and need to look at their individual response to a varied schedule. If it's not broken don't try to fix it." The comment is very thoughtful and absolutely true as well, and there is no textbook on how to manage patients' medications because there are literally hundreds to thousands of variables that can affect medication management. For me personally, I'm going to lean in and attempt to investigate how and why this patient ended up on twice daily pioglitazone and a once weekly oxybutynin patch. If the primary provider has no idea (or can't remember) and the patient doesn't know why either, I'm in the camp that is probably going to attempt to take some risk to reduce medication burden. I would consolidate the pioglitazone and monitor blood sugars as well as closely assess the patient's urinary symptoms and recommend a trial hold of the oxybutynin patch to minimize anticholinergic burden going forward. If the patient is adamant that the medications are working well, are well tolerated, and have improved their diabetes, urinary symptoms, and overall wellbeing, of course I wouldn't suggest any changes.

I wanted to use this comment to demonstrate that it can be challenging to address medication related problems and even more challenging to address them when everything is going fine with our patients. I believe the "If It's Not Broke, Don't Fix It" philosophy is one of the major culprits that leads to polypharmacy. At what point does too many medications actually become "too many medications"? If the patient is on 52 medications, is that too many? If they feel perfectly fine on 52 medications and are doing well, should we not reduce or change anything? If a patient is on two medications that do the same thing but are doing fine, should we leave it alone? Every patient brings a whole set of new circumstances that has to be considered. "What is polypharmacy?" depends upon the provider, depends upon the patient, and is a question that each healthcare professional has to find a comfort level with.

For me, I work primarily in geriatrics and when I hear, "if it's not broke, don't fix it", I can feel polypharmacy creeping in. It's a mindset that is easy to have, but I do not believe it is the best mindset for the majority of my patients. Notice how I said "majority", not all patients. Healthcare professionals disagree, and I would make the argument that if there is no disagreement, there's no critical thinking happening. I have had the unique opportunity to make recommendations to well over 100+ different providers/healthcare professionals. While I feel I do my job in a consistent manner, there are providers that agree with nearly everything I suggest, and there are providers that disagree with many of my recommendations, and I'm ok with that. What's your philosophy?

Respiratory Med List Review

Current Medications:
Albuterol nebulizer four times daily
Mirtazapine 30 mg at bedtime
Prednisone 10 mg twice daily
Tylenol prn
Oxygen 2 liters
Spiriva one daily
Pravachol 40 mg daily
Advair 250/50 mg one twice daily
Lidocaine patch 1 q12 hours on/off prn
K-Dur 20 mEq three times daily
Aspirin 81 mg daily
Multivitamin one daily
Lasix 40 mg twice daily
Protonix 40 mg daily
Diltiazem 180 mg daily
Ativan 0.5 mg prn

My top two priorities:
1. Pretty obvious to see from the meds that this patient has some significant respiratory issues. Between Advair, Spiriva, albuterol, oxygen, and (likely) oral prednisone – this patient obviously struggles in that department. It is always important to try to minimize systemic prednisone if possible, so I would like to know if that's a chronic dose or a short term burst. If chronic prednisone is necessary, osteoporosis amongst other things should be

assessed/treated as appropriate (i.e. Vitamin D, Bisphosphonate).
2. Decent doses of furosemide/potassium, so I'd make sure the electrolytes/kidney function look okay.

Clinical Medication Review

Current Medications:
Amlodipine 10 mg daily
Aspirin 81 mg daily
Vitamin D3 2,000 units daily
Colace 100 mg daily
Avodart 0.5 mg daily
Lasix 40 mg daily
Percocet 2 tablets after breakfast
Cozaar 50 mg daily
Metoprolol XL 25 mg daily
Multivitamin 1 tablet daily
Prilosec 20 mg daily
Potassium chloride 20 mEq every Monday
Ranitidine 150 mg daily
Zocor 20 mg daily
Tramadol 50 mg every morning
Maxzide 37.5/25 tablet daily

Both omeprazole and ranitidine are being utilized here. I would like to look into the GI history and assess if both are necessary. Judging by this patient's other meds, he/she is not at very high risk for GI bleeding as only on low dose aspirin, but again I would need to investigate history further.

Plenty of BP meds noted, and I would suspect edema or CHF history. I would like to dig into furosemide and triamterene/hydrochlorothiazide (Maxzide) history to assess if both are necessary. Remember that Maxzide is a combo of diuretics and does work differently from furosemide, but when trying to tackle polypharmacy, this might be a place to look into further. Also remember that Maxzide contains triamterene, a potassium sparing diuretic, which might be helping to stabilize potassium levels as both the furosemide and hydrochlorothiazide (in Maxzide) can bring potassium down. Duplicate opioids (tramadol and Percocet) need some investigating as well!

Quinine for Leg Cramps

Current Medications:
Acetaminophen 500mg 1-2 q 4-6 h prn
Alprazolam 0.25mg at bedtime prn
Atorvastatin 20mg daily
Calcium Carbonate w/Vitamin D 600mg twice daily
Coreg 12.5mg twice daily
Cod Liver Oil 1 capsule daily
Vitamin B12 1000mcg IM/month
Digoxin 125mcg daily
Duo Neb treatment twice daily
Enalapril 5mg twice daily
Flonase 2 sprays to each nostril/day prn
Glucosamine 500mg 2 twice daily
Ipratropium Albuterol Rescue Inhaler three times daily prn
Furosemide 40mg twice daily
Metformin 500mg ½ tab daily
Mucinex 600mg twice daily
Nitroglycerine SL prn
Potassium Chloride 20mEq twice daily
Pulmicort neb treatment twice daily
Quinine 325mg at bedtime prn
Simethicone 80mg 1-2 tab daily
Warfarin 3mg daily

Quinine for leg cramps has a boxed warning in the U.S. due to potential for serious side effects like arrhythmias and thrombocytopenia. In studies, it has been shown to be ineffective for leg cramps in addition to the risks of adverse effects. Occasionally, I do see it used. I'd focus on trying to identify if the cramps are due to another identifiable cause like an electrolyte imbalance (potassium, magnesium, etc.), which we can check labs for (patient is on furosemide). If the pain is more muscle soreness versus cramping, certainly the statin should be ruled out. I might be inclined to see if a trial of scheduled acetaminophen would work if the patient is having pain at night. Seeing the alprazolam at night makes me think the patient has trouble sleeping, another reason to rule out the pain issue, but certainly we need to assess this with the patient.

Medication List Review – Erythromycin

Current Medications:
Imdur 30 mg daily
Metoprolol tartrate 12.5 daily
Atorvastatin 20mg at bedtime
Lorazepam 0.5 mg twice daily
Lexapro 20 mg daily
Aricept 10 mg daily
Namenda XR 28 mg daily
Abilify 2 mg daily
Erythromycin 125 mg three times daily
Pepcid 40 mg daily
Acetaminophen 650 mg twice daily
Duonebs four times daily
FA 1 mg daily
Calcium Vitamin D 500 mg/400 units twice daily

MVI daily
Senna S as needed
Imodium as needed

The first thing I want you to remember whenever you see an order for erythromycin is that it has a ton of drug interactions. Whenever we start, increase or decrease this medication, it can have ramifications on the concentrations of other medications.

I will highlight a couple possible interactions; erythromycin can increase aripiprazole (Abilify) concentrations. Here's a case where dose really makes a difference. While it is a legitimate concern, my concern would be much higher if this patient was on 30 mg of aripiprazole daily versus the current 2 mg order. Atorvastatin concentrations can also be increased due to the erythromycin, so this is something we need to monitor and be thinking about.

The other question I'd have with the erythromycin is why are we using it? I've seen this type of dosing before and would likely suspect chronic use not for an infection, but for GI motility. I'm not a big fan of using this due to all the interactions erythromycin can cause, but it might be the only option depending upon the case.

Medication List Review – Allergies

<u>Current Medications:</u>
Metoprolol 50 mg twice daily
Flecainide 100 mg twice daily
Zocor 40 mg at bedtime
Buspirone 15 mg AM 30 mg PM
Remeron 30 mg at bedtime
Pantoprazole 40 mg daily

Acetaminophen 650 mg as needed
Loratadine 20 mg daily
Fluticasone nasal spray prn

Here's my breakdown: Knowing your doses is important, and the obvious medication with an abnormally high dose is loratadine. Usual dosing is 10 mg daily. Given the higher dose and fluticasone order, I would suspect a very substantial allergy or rhinitis history. We could look at scheduling fluticasone depending on current control of symptoms.

I would also suspect pretty significant anxiety/mental health issues as this patient is on both mirtazapine (Remeron) and buspirone (Buspar). This could use much further investigation as well. It is always important to remember the key characteristic of buspirone versus the benzodiazepines for anxiety: Buspirone generally takes a significant amount of time to start working (i.e. maybe weeks) which differs greatly from the benzo's (like lorazepam, alprazolam, etc.). Hence, you shouldn't ever see an as needed order for buspirone, but I frequently see them for benzo's. An obvious disadvantage of the benzodiazepines is that they have sedative/confusion side effects that can be particularly troubling in the elderly. Another obvious disadvantage of benzo's is they are controlled substances in the US.

Vital signs like pulse and blood pressure are going to be very important with this patient being on flecainide and metoprolol.

I also can't help but wonder about possible antiplatelet therapy like aspirin. The patient certainly could've had some issues with bleeding or other problems, but this is something that should be investigated with the use of metoprolol, flecainide, and simvastatin (Zocor).

Medication List Case Review

Current Medications:
 Tylenol 650 mg twice daily
Allopurinol 100 mg daily
Amiodarone 200 mg every other day
Norvasc 5 mg twice daily
Aspirin 81 mg daily
Lipitor 10 mg daily
Fibercon, one tablet daily
Vitamin D3 1000 units daily
Plavix 75 mg daily
Doxazosin 2 mg at bedtime
Neurontin 600 mg three times daily
Glyburide 2.5 mg daily
Hydralazine 100 mg three times daily
Imdur 60 mg in the afternoon, 120 mg in the morning

Hydralazine and Imdur doses are pretty substantial, leading me to believe that this individual has significant cardiac/hypertension issues. This patient is also on amiodarone, amlodipine, aspirin, clopidogrel, atorvastatin, and doxazosin. Blood pressure monitoring will be very important. Remember that amiodarone has some funky side effects to monitor for.

It appears from the med list that this patient has diabetes with the glyburide Rx. I'd investigate why he isn't on an ACE or ARB especially since he most likely has significant issues with blood pressure. If he hasn't been on an ACE or ARB for some reason (allergy, contraindication, or adverse drug reaction), I'd look at a possible transition from the doxazosin unless the doxazosin is being used for BPH and hypertension.

There are likely some pain issues with scheduled acetaminophen (likely gabapentin at a decent sized dose as well). I would suspect a gout diagnosis with the allopurinol Rx.

I'd try to investigate why amlodipine is twice daily. Some providers prefer twice daily especially if having variable BP's, but it might be a place where we can minimize pill burden.

Antiplatelet Therapy

Current Medications:
Celexa 20 mg nightly
Famotidine 20 mg daily
Imdur 60 mg daily
Lantus 70 units nightly
Lasix 20 mg daily
Levothyroxine 25 mcg daily
Metoprolol 12.5 mg daily
Morphine p.r.n. chest pain
Senna 1 tab every day
Simvastatin 40 mg nightly
Vitamin D 2000 units daily
Namenda 10 mg twice daily
Triamcinolone cream twice daily
Carbidopa/levodopa 25/100 three times daily
NovoLog 10 units three times daily
Acetaminophen 650 mg three times daily

The morphine dose certainly needs to be clarified, and we might as well ask how frequently it is used for chest pain.

Along with the potential for chest pain and a significant number of cardiac type medications, it is pretty suspicious that this patient is not on an antiplatelet medication of any kind.

The other point I will mention is that this patient is on a fairly substantial dose of insulin. We need to pay close attention to blood sugars and any abnormal symptoms as this patient likely has dementia being on the Namenda. Hypoglycemia identification can often be a challenge in dementia and polypharmacy.

Enoxaparin (Lovenox), NSAIDs and Bleed Risk

Discharge Medications:
Amlodipine 5 mg daily
Aspirin 325 mg daily
Vitamin B12 1000 mcg by mouth daily
Lovenox 30 mg subq twice daily for DVT prophylaxis.
Flaxseed two tabs daily
Neurontin 900 mg twice daily
Lasix 20 mg daily
Glucosamine two tabs daily
Indocin 25 mg three times daily
Combivent one puff four times daily
Losartan 50 mg daily
Thiamine 100 mg daily
Acetaminophen 650 mg every 4 hours prn
DuoNeb every 4 hours prn
Nitroglycerin sublingual 0.4 mg prn
Oxycodone 5 to 10 mg every 4 hours prn
Seroquel 12.5 mg at bedtime.

It is always important to take a look at the enoxaparin dose to make sure it is correct and that we have an end date in mind when using it for prophylaxis. I'm also going to look at the indomethacin with the enoxaparin as this patient will be at high risk for GI bleeding. She is on aspirin as well. GI protection should be considered with close monitoring of hemoglobin/platelets while on the enoxaparin especially.

There are so many things to investigate, but that quetiapine just screams at me as I've seen antipsychotics used so many times for acute delirium situations and then left on board long term. I'm going to try to investigate why this patient was put on this medication and see if we can possibly get rid of it. With the use of thiamine, this patient could very well have a history of alcoholism, something to dig into as well in the patient history.

Medication Review: Hypertension

Current Medications:

Amlodipine 5 mg daily
Aspirin 81 mg daily
Clonidine 0.1 mg at bedtime and 0.2 mg qAM
Coumadin daily
Cranberry capsules 600 mg daily
Ferrous sulfate 325 mg twice daily
FloraQ capsule daily
Gabapentin 300 mg four times daily
Hydrocodone-APAP 5/325 mg tablet every four hours prn
Potassium 40 mEq daily
Losartan 100 mg daily
Macrobid 100 mg daily
Metoprolol 12.5 mg twice daily
MiraLax 17 g daily

Multivitamin daily
Omeprazole 40 mg daily
Senokot S tablet twice daily
Simvastatin 10 mg daily
Tamsulosin 0.8 mg daily
Torsemide 40 mg in the morning 20 mg in the afternoon
Tramadol 50 mg three times daily
Vitamin E 400 units daily

This medication list tells me the patient has high blood pressure. Amlodipine, clonidine, losartan, metoprolol, as well as torsemide and tamsulosin have the potential to bring the blood pressure down. It certainly looks like this is a case where we would need to monitor blood pressure closely. Tamsulosin is more selective for the prostate, but it can still have an effect on the vessels.

On the positive side, there isn't any duplication in the classes of antihypertensives being used. I don't see any notorious medications that cause or worsen hypertension. From the medications, I'm also guessing that this patient has a history of anemia (on iron supplementation). We need to always assess ongoing use of iron as it can be problematic especially in the elderly (GI side effects, constipating, drug interactions, etc.). If the anemia is significant, we will need to continually assess the warfarin use closely as well.

I would suspect this is an elderly patient, so I would also be looking closely at kidney function. The nitrofurantoin is especially something important I'd be checking out. There are plenty of other labs and vitals that need to be monitored; electrolytes, kidney function, pulses, CBC, and INR to list a few.

Assessment of pain would be an important factor as well as this can play a role in contributing to elevated blood pressure. The regimen seems a little bizarre with scheduled tramadol and prn hydrocodone/APAP.

Why the vitamin E, and is cranberry (usually for UTI prevention) of benefit when already taking nitrofurantoin!?!?

Clinical Pharmacy Thought Process

Current Medications:
DuoNebs four times daily
Fosamax 70 mg weekly
Amlodipine 5 mg daily
Amoxicillin/clavulanate 875 mg twice daily
Aspirin 81 mg daily
Amoxicillin 875 mg daily
Aspirin 81 mg daily
Benadryl 25 mg every 6 hours as needed
CPAP nighttime use
Calcium with Vitamin D 500/200 units daily
Vitamin D 1,000 units daily
Cozaar 12.5 mg daily
Cymbalta 60 mg daily
Gabapentin 800 mg four times daily
Miralax 17 grams daily as needed
Potassium 40 mEq four times daily
Oxycodone 2.5 mg every 4 hours as needed
Senokot S as needed
Spiriva 18 mcg daily
Symbicort 160 mcg daily
Synthroid 188 mcg daily
Torsemide 50 mg twice daily
Tramadol 50 mg every 6 hours

Tylenol 650 mg every 6 hours
Zaroxolyn 2.5 mg as needed for weight gain of 3 pounds in a day

I'm going to highlight a couple of things that I would be looking at closely. The first thing I notice was the duplication amoxicillin/Augmentin – likely an error in transcribing, but something that needs to be looked at for sure.

Going down further on the list, I notice pretty substantial doses that we should keep a watchful eye on depending upon age, kidney function and other factors. Gabapentin is at a fairly big dose of 800 mg four times daily, and that especially concerns me as this patient is on 2 diuretics. Remember that gabapentin and amlodipine are two common medications that can contribute to edema. I would likely guess the gabapentin is being used for neuropathy type pain (duloxetine as well), but I can only speculate.

The other big dose that you need to have a healthy respect for is potassium 40 mEq four times daily. This is a very big dose of potassium – it may likely be very necessary given the significant diuretic use but something that should be monitored closely at a minimum. Metolazone as needed makes me a little nervous as well, not necessarily that it shouldn't be done, but you could anticipate that if the patient takes this frequently or not at all, electrolytes (especially potassium) could certainly fluctuate. Depending upon diagnosis and other considerations, this patient may be a candidate to consider spironolactone to help raise potassium and potentially reduce the need for the high dose potassium supplementation. Increasing losartan might also help with this, but again we need to check out lots of different factors to make that judgment.

Clinical Med List Review – Primidone

A 78 year old male was recently admitted to the hospital with a fall and likely hip fracture. He has had some lethargy and confusion as well. Previous falls have been noted.

Current Medications:
Calcium and Vitamin D twice daily
Proscar 5 mg daily
Tamsulosin 0.4 mg daily
Primidone 500 mg four times daily
Aspirin 325 mg daily
Enalapril 5 mg daily
Tylenol 500 mg twice daily as needed
Senna 1-2 tabs as needed
Artificial tears as needed
Percocet 5/325 1-2 tablets as needed for pain
Gabapentin 100 mg at night
Propranolol 80 mg twice daily
Benadryl 50 mg at night for sleep
Metoprolol 25 mg twice daily

There are quite a few possible concerns to note with this medication list. One of the major problems of polypharmacy that I see is that things just have a much greater risk of being overlooked. If you have a patient on two medications, it is pretty easy to rule out medication related issues in a minute or two. When patients are on 10, 20, 30+, things just slip through the cracks.

The first thing I'm going to pull out here is the terrifying dose of primidone. If this is a medication you don't know much about, I'd suggest you take a look at it. This is a ridiculously high dose that should scare the pants off you. I can't even recall a dose half that size in any other patient I've seen before. I would suspect the diagnosis is essential tremor as usually that's the diagnosis, but it is an old antiepileptic so it could be utilized for seizures. In any case, this dose likely needs to be reduced, or we need to at least check a level with a phenobarbital level as primidone is converted to phenobarb in the body.

Second: Two beta blockers. Propranolol makes me lean toward primidone being used for tremors, but I would have to verify that with the past medical history.

Third: You can notice the possible "trigger" medications as I call them. These are medications that likely are treating side effects of other medications (prescribing cascade). We have Senna, Artificial Tears, as well as medications for BPH/urinary retention. Remember that these symptoms/medications scream anticholinergic effects, likely related to the scheduled diphenhydramine at bedtime in this case.

PERSONAL STORIES

What can a Clinical Pharmacist Bring to the Table?

I feel like I'm always trying to educate folks what a clinical pharmacist can provide to patients, nurses, physicians, a healthcare team, or institution. Ever since I was accepted into pharmacy school, I feel like I've been hearing about MTM (medication therapy management) and clinical pharmacy, and when you talk to virtually anyone outside of the world of pharmacy, no one has a clue what you're talking about.

I do work in rural areas, so maybe that does skew my experience. Maybe I'm not very good at selling our services? Or even worse, maybe we pharmacists have a bad product? I'm biased but the second question isn't true.
A question asked by an administrator at an assisted living really got me frustrated, but it really did cause me to think. The question was: Why would we need someone else to review a medication list when the doctor and nurses already do that? In hindsight, it is a really good question and one I should've thought about a long time ago. When I put myself in the shoes of that administrator, the question is very legitimate, and I feel like that is the giant hurdle I face every day in trying to prove the value of what I do. At the time, I had no response and ceded that she wasn't interested in what I would provide. I could certainly list studies and case reports that prove the value, cost savings, improvement of health related outcomes, satisfaction and on and on, but to be honest, that's boring.

That question of what we do differently as clinical pharmacists has stuck with me for a few years now, and

I'm finally gaining some perspective on that question. Just put yourself in the mindset of the administrator who knows very little about pharmacy, and you will come to this conclusion. Pharmacists don't do anything differently. (I'm sure all my pharmacist friends are up in arms right now!) Does the physician or nurse review the medication list? Does the physician or nurse review appropriate labs? Does the physician or nurse take into account patient concerns, objective and subjective information? All the answers are yes which leads me to my conclusion that clinical pharmacists don't do anything different than an attending primary care provider or nurse taking care of a patient. Here's the insight. While we don't physically do anything different from a physician when reviewing medications, clinical pharmacists use a different tool. We have a different lens that we look through when assessing patients, and that's the beauty of all of us working together.

Let me explain. Where a nurse might see a patient failing in the end stages of dementia, I see an inappropriate increase in phenytoin causing toxicity. Where a physician might see a new diagnosis of dry eyes, I see a patient on duplicate anticholinergic drugs. Where a physician might see a patient with worsening CHF, I see a patient that was just recently started on celecoxib for pain. Where a nurse might see worsening symptoms of gout, I see that hydrochlorothiazide for blood pressure was recently initiated. Where a physician discontinues rifampin for osteomyelitis, I see a very significant drug interaction requiring additional monitoring in a patient on warfarin. Our pharmacist lens allows us to focus on medication related problems that put our patients at risk of adverse effects, poor outcomes, drug interactions, hospitalizations, or worse.

What is it Like in a Long Term Care Facility?

I can't say thank you enough to all the aides, nurses and others who help take care of those who cannot care for themselves.

This has really been in and out my mind the last few weeks, and I can't quite shake it. I was working at a facility, sitting at one of the nurses' stations and was watching a worker absolutely loving on a resident, treating her as if she was their own flesh and blood. Being outside the ring of direct resident care, I don't get to pay a ton of attention to the residents but enjoy the time I do get to share with them. The way the staff member was treating this resident should've been a training video for how to treat people with kindness, love, and respect.

Then I almost got a little choked up and felt sadness overtake me. I wasn't sad for the resident's situation, or the difficult job that the worker has, but because I knew that this would never be a headline in a newspaper, or on the evening news, or a viral video everyone sends to their friends. So to those not familiar with the ins and outs of nursing home care, I'd like to challenge you to think a little differently the next time you see an article about neglect, abuse, or theft and just understand the headlines you see are not the norm.

Medication Mistakes can be Stepping Stones to Better Care

Ever made a mistake? I have. I will never forget that feeling – it's awful.

I was reviewing a patient's medication list and noted that the patient was struggling with the costs of their medications. I was a fairly recent graduate at the time, and the patient was taking atorvastatin (brand name Lipitor at that time) at a dose of 10 mg. I suggested that we change it to simvastatin (Zocor) 20 mg which was generic and much cheaper. This is a recommendation I had certainly made before. What I failed to realize was that this patient had an intolerance to simvastatin that was on their allergy list. (By the way, this is why we have multiple checks in place to prevent one person's mistake from getting to the patient.) I flat out missed it. I remember coming across it at a later date (which I'm very thankful to be able to learn from this without patient harm), and I found that a wonderful nurse had caught my error and prevented a negative outcome. When I went to thank her for catching the error and saving me, she was totally oblivious and could hardly even remember it. Medication errors happen because we are imperfect people trying to serve our patients perfectly. I tell you this story because it's real, and it happens. We all must learn from our own mistakes, as well as from the mistakes of others to continuously improve the quality and safety of our care. Paraphrasing Vince Lombardi, "Relentlessly pursue perfection, and along the way you'll catch excellence." To the nurse who I'm sure doesn't remember this story by now, thank you. We are all in this together.

Witty Old Man Seeking Viagra

We all know that Viagra (sildenafil) can be used for erectile dysfunction, but this elderly patient was seeking it for an off label use.

This gentleman was frequently asking his doctor and the nurses that worked with him if he could get "a little bit" of

Viagra. He was elderly, a fall risk, and on a bunch of blood pressure medications that certainly wouldn't mix well with the Viagra, and obviously the doctor couldn't help but think what he'd use it for anyway. Finally after getting tired of the questioning, the doctor broke down and asked the elderly man what he wanted the Viagra for, and also why he was always insistent that he only needed "a little bit". Obviously the doctor was expecting some sort of perverted answer. The man spouted back, "I only need a little bit to keep me from peeing on my shoes."

I'm Thankful for Great People!

A few months back, I had this enlightening interaction with a nursing home resident. I was working at a nurses' station and this elderly gentleman strolls by in his wheel chair, telling me I must be a student (probably because I look like I'm 12). I said no, I'm actually a pharmacist. He looked very confused. I tried to ask him how his day was going, and again he looked confused.

At this point, I was starting to think that he most likely had some form of dementia. Then he asked me, "How are the crops looking out there and is anyone out in the field?" Seeing an opening, I said there are some combines out working on wheat. "Did you grow up on a farm?" he asked. I said to him, "You probably won't believe me, but I did. How about you?" He simply replied, "All my life." At this point, I was starting to figure out that he was a little more with it than I had initially given him credit. Then he asked me, "Why aren't you farming?" and I said that I just decided to take a different path. At this point, he was looking at me like I had a "third eye" to quote one of my colleagues. You could tell what he was thinking, why would anyone not want to farm if they had the chance?

Then, you could tell he was starting to put it together as he said, "You have brothers don't you?" I said I have three older brothers. "I bet one of them farms," he said. "You got it," I told him. The world was right again in his mind. I thoroughly enjoy my time with the elderly. It is one of the aspects of my work that makes it truly special.

Give More, Complain Less = Unbelievable Opportunity

Before I began my 2nd full time career as an educator online, I found myself complaining about others more often than I would like. Why didn't this nurse know this? Why didn't this doctor know that? What was that pharmacist thinking? I somehow did a 180 with those complaints into a direct question to myself; what was I doing about it? The truth to that answer cut deep. The truth was, I was doing bits and pieces to help educate, but there was zero doubt in my mind that I could give more and complain less.

The reality of giving more has taken me to a place in my professional career that I never could've dreamed. I've had wonderful colleagues contribute great content, been offered various interviews, had opportunities to guest post on blogs, had some of the most kind people give words of encouragement and praise, been mentioned in a national journal, and had my cases shared literally to thousands of healthcare professionals spanning over 100 countries, but I will never forget the day it got real.

In September 2014, I received an email from a reporter asking my thoughts on a medication (Namenda) related news story. Yes, my thoughts. This reporter was not from my local hometown paper (no offense Northern Star). This reporter was from the Wall Street Journal. Yes, that Wall

Street FREAKIN Journal! Pardon my language. The newspaper with the highest circulation in the US! I was humbled beyond belief and thrilled to have this unique opportunity. One tweet out of thousands gave me this chance, but I couldn't help but think why me versus the thousands of other quality healthcare professionals out there? Other than dumb luck, the only explanation I have for this has been my change in attitude to giving more. Without social media and blogging, there is no chance I'd have this opportunity at even the end of my career, much less in the earlier stages. Honored is the best word I can come up with, but that doesn't do it justice.

PRESCRIBING CASCADE

Dose and Drug Matter

An elderly patient was on cetirizine (Zyrtec) 10 mg at bedtime for allergies and was also on oxybutynin (Ditropan) 15 mg three times daily for urinary incontinence. Oxybutynin is one of those classic older anticholinergic medications that isn't so great in the elderly (noted to be in the Beer's criteria). This patient was experiencing significant dry mouth and dry eyes. The physician was concerned with the cetirizine causing the anticholinergic symptoms (my assumption was the oxybutynin was overlooked). I was taught a couple of ways to remember a few of the major anticholinergic effects. Some use the acronym SLUDs – Meaning you CANNOT Salivate, Lacrimate, Urinate, or Defecate. Others use "can't spit, see, pee or poop (enter explicative)" to describe anticholinergic effects. CNS effects like confusion and fall risk are also problematic with anticholinergic effects especially in the elderly.

Keeping an eye out for "trigger" medications that treat these symptoms is really important (i.e. artificial tears or saliva, alpha blockers like tamsulosin due to urinary retention). In this case, if incontinence was well controlled or if the drug was ineffective, the oxybutynin would likely be the medication I would be strongly advocating to decrease as 45 mg total daily dose is a very steep dose compared to the anticholinergic activity that 10 mg of cetirizine would have.

Anticholinergics can Worsen BPH

An 85 year old male with a recent operation for a knee replacement was discharged on hydrocodone/APAP 5/325mg 1-2 tabs every four hours as needed as well as hydroxyzine (Vistaril) 25-50 mg every six hours as needed for pain management. Within a couple days of significant prn use for the pain, the patient was experiencing constipation issues that were easily managed with Senna-S 2 tablets daily. After about 5-7 days, this patient began to have worsening urinary retention and was placed on tamsulosin (Flomax) 0.4 mg daily to help treat the retention. The following day, the retention was getting even worse and a Foley catheter had to be placed. This gentleman did have a history of BPH and retention, and here's a perfect demonstration why anticholinergics (hydroxyzine) in the elderly should be avoided or at least be minimized. This patient was using the 50 mg dose as often as he could which was certainly worsening the urinary retention.

Amiodarone

A patient had begun to experience some shortness of breath especially with walking and other physical activity. He was diagnosed with COPD and was placed on a long acting anticholinergic medication tiotropium (Spiriva) to help alleviate those symptoms, as well as Duonebs (short acting beta agonist with short acting anticholinergic) on an as needed basis. Symptoms continued to worsen, and a long acting corticosteroid plus long acting beta agonist (Advair or Symbicort type medication) was initiated to help treat the respiratory issues. This gradual decline in lung function led the healthcare team to investigate the possibility that amiodarone was causing this.

Amiodarone has a black box warning due to its ability to cause pulmonary fibrosis. This patient was referred to a cardiologist who determined the risk of this side effect was greater than any potential benefit from the drug, so amiodarone was discontinued.

Dementia Medication Case

In a case I came across a while back, it was a classic prescribing cascade example. For those of you who've never heard this term, it essentially means treating side effects of one medication with another medication. Rivastigmine (Exelon patches) had been initiated for dementia and was subsequently increased after a month or two. A couple weeks after the increase in dose, it was evident that this patient was having some GI symptoms as ondansetron (Zofran) was added to treat symptoms of nausea and stomach upset.

Hydrochlorothiazide and Elevated Uric Acid

A patient was being treated for hypertension. He had isolated systolic high blood pressure. Systolic blood pressures (BP) were running in the 150-160 range. Hydrochlorothiazide was the drug that was chosen to help treat the elevated BP. The dosing was 25 mg daily. After a couple of weeks, the blood pressures were lower by about 10-15 points, and follow up kidney labs and electrolytes were stable. Hydrochlorothiazide is a "thiazide" diuretic, real original I know. About a month later, this patient had an acute gout flare, and a uric acid level was checked and elevated. Allopurinol was added to treat the elevation in uric acid. What was missed, however, was that hydrochlorothiazide can have this adverse effect of causing uric acid levels to increase.

Gabapentin and Kidney Function Changes

An elderly patient had been on a dose of gabapentin (Neurontin) 600 mg three times daily for peripheral neuropathy. Over time, the patient's kidney function declined, and he was diagnosed with chronic kidney disease.

The family had begun to notice that the patient was becoming more lethargic and dizzy. The patient had also made the comment that he felt "snowed" at times. Meclizine was added as needed to help treat the dizziness, and the team decided to monitor the other symptoms at this time. The peripheral neuropathy was well managed with no noted pain stated by the patient.

Because of the decline in kidney function, the previous dose of gabapentin was now inappropriate especially in this case secondary to the noted adverse effects. Gabapentin is primarily eliminated from the body through the kidney. Gabapentin was reduced, and the patient's symptoms did resolve. The meclizine added for dizziness was also eventually discontinued as we didn't have any side effects to treat anymore.

Allopurinol – Drug Induced Rash

A 78 year old male was on a hefty list of medications. The major issue to resolve was a rash that had started about 3-4 weeks ago and was spreading nearly all over the body. I was asked to help out with the case by looking over the meds. There had already been a couple of meds held to rule out the possibility of the rash being drug induced. In medication management, the first place to look when new symptoms happen is the changes that had been made previous to the new symptoms. In this case, furosemide (Lasix) had been increased and sertraline (Zoloft) had been started within the last few months. Both had been held for over a week, and it was felt that the rash was not improving. At this point, the primary provider did not feel as if it was medication related and was searching for another diagnosis and dermatology involvement.

Not so fast. What was noted was that this patient had chronic kidney disease (CKD), and the kidney function had been changing over the previous few years. The baseline creatinine had gone from about 1.2-1.5 range and was now consistently above 2 mg/dL. Estimated GFR had dropped between 20-30 ml/min. Amongst the massive medication list was a seemingly innocent dose of allopurinol 300 mg daily. Remember that allopurinol is cleared by the kidney and with the worsening kidney function, this drug was sure to be at higher concentrations in the body than it was years ago. The allopurinol was held and a low dose of colchicine 0.3 mg daily was initiated without issue. (Remember that colchicine needs to be dose adjusted for kidney function as well.) The rash began to resolve over time and all was well again!

Causes of GI Irritation and PPI Use

This is an example I see all too often. A patient gets started on a medication that is known to cause GI side effects like nausea, heartburn, or GI ulcer. In my practice, a few classic examples of meds that can cause stomach irritation or other GI issues are NSAIDs, prednisone, metformin, and acetylcholinesterase inhibitors. A recent case I had was where a patient was starting on a prednisone burst for arthritis for a period of time and was having some GI side effects (obviously from the prednisone in my mind). While on prednisone the resident was experiencing some heartburn and nausea. A PPI (omeprazole) was subsequently added and symptoms resolved. The moral of this story is that the prednisone was later tapered off and discontinued, so do you think she would still need the PPI?

Trazodone use for Insomnia

A 68 year old female was having difficulty with some anxiety throughout the day, but more problematic to the patient was that she could not sleep at night. Multiple different non-drug interventions were tried, but none seemed to make any difference. Trazodone was finally prescribed, and insomnia did improve but only minimally. This particular patient was also on levothyroxine (Synthroid) 75 mcg daily for treatment of hypothyroidism. Due to the anxiety and insomnia continuing despite the trazodone order, a TSH was finally ordered. The TSH was significantly suppressed at 0.05 indicating an over supplementation of levothyroxine. The dose was reduced. When the patient's TSH was finally within the normal range, symptoms of anxiety and insomnia greatly improved, and the trazodone was eventually discontinued.

Overactive Bladder and UTI Case

I've come across this type of situation a few different times. A patient gets diagnosed with a UTI and is started on an antibiotic. Pretty standard situation that happens frequently and not a big deal. It was noted that there was an increase in frequency of urination, a pretty common occurrence when individuals have a UTI especially in the geriatric population. The part that drives me crazy is the individual gets put on a medication to help with the frequency (solifenacin or Vesicare) the very same day that the antibiotic is started. The UTI resolves and the patient gets left on the drug for frequency! Why not wait until the UTI has resolved to address and treat frequent urination symptoms if actually necessary? They weren't on the solifenacin before the UTI, so would they need it after successful treatment?

Drug Induced Weight Loss – An Order That Should Sound an Alarm

While in much of the population a controlled, planned weight loss can be a good thing, it cannot be a good thing sometimes as well. Drug induced weight loss (especially in the elderly) does happen, and you need to be able to identify it!

If you ever see an order for Ensure or other nutritional supplements, just stop for one second and think about it. What does this order mean? This order likely means that the patient receiving the supplement is struggling with weight loss, nutrition, and/or appetite issues. There are boatloads of medications that can contribute to weight loss, and recognition of orders like this can help you identify that patients may be having adverse effects from their medications.

There are also many disease states that if undertreated or over treated can cause weight loss. Stop and take a look at their medications and diagnoses; you may find that they don't need a supplement but need to have their medications and conditions assessed for drug induced weight loss. Too much levothyroxine, digoxin, stimulants, and acetylcholinesterase inhibitors are a few examples of medications with the potential to cause weight loss. Address potential side effects first before searching for alternatives to help treat their weight loss!

Colchicine Can Cause Significant Diarrhea

An 88 year old gentleman was having a difficult time with management of gout. He was on chronic allopurinol therapy and had to use frequent as needed NSAIDs for repeat flares. Steroid bursts also had to be used to treat acute flares. Remember that there are some medications that can contribute to gout symptoms by elevating uric acid (thiazide diuretics and niacin are a couple that come to mind). These had been ruled out in this case. Because of the repeated flares, the patient was placed on colchicine 0.6 mg twice daily. After about a week of therapy, the patient was started on loperamide (Imodium) for diarrhea. The diarrhea did not resolve, so cholestyramine (Questran) was added and improvement was noted. Colchicine can cause very high rates of diarrhea. This is also a pretty steep dose of colchicine in an 88 year old.

I'd like to explore other options to help manage the gout to try to avoid the colchicine. Another consideration is to decrease the dose to try to minimize these side effects while still adequately treating the condition. One last point (as there are times where treating side effects may be necessary if the team/patient deem appropriate) going back to our case: It is critical to identify those medications that may not be effective and stop them! In this case, was the loperamide effective?

Stimulant Use In Adults

<u>Current Medications:</u>
Tylenol every 6 hours prn
DuoNebs three times a day
Aspirin 81 mg daily
Clonazepam 0.5 mg three times daily
Digoxin 0.125 mg daily
Senokot S twice daily with meals
Furosemide 20 mg daily
Glyburide 5 mg twice daily
Isosorbide mononitrate 30 mg daily
Levothyroxine 50 mcg daily
Lisinopril 20 mg daily
Ritalin 10 mg twice daily at 8:00 and noon
Metoprolol succinate 50 mg daily
Mirtazapine 30 mg at bedtime
Mirapex 0.25 mg daily at bedtime
Venlafaxine 150 mg daily
Warfarin 4 mg daily
Docusate 100 mg daily as needed for constipation
Hydrocodone acetaminophen 5/325 mg one tablet
Milk of Magnesia prn
Nitroglycerin prn

I do see methylphenidate (Ritalin) used in adults from time to time, and this medication case study certainly identifies some issues that methylphenidate could be complicating.

Let's dig into this medication list, and I will give you my top three things to consider. When we get a med list like this, it can often be a challenge as to what to prioritize first. Patient specifics are certainly going to guide you as to what is most important as well, but I feel that reviewing a medication list serves as a great educational tool.

This is likely an adult patient going by the medication list, which leads me to my first concern in using the methylphenidate. He apparently has some significant cardiac/hypertension issues based on the med list as well as potentially anxiety (clonazepam) and possibly insomnia (mirtazapine use at bedtime). Both of these can be exacerbated by the methylphenidate. It looks as if this is a possible case of upper and downer type medications combating each other. This needs to be investigated further.

Monitoring of vital signs is going to be very important looking at the number of meds that can lower blood pressure in addition to the above mentioned methylphenidate which can increase it. Blood sugars and pulses will need to be followed closely as well given the glyburide use and metoprolol/digoxin combination.

In addition to vitals, there are plenty of labs to check; TSH, INR, CBC, BMP to name a few due to levothyroxine, warfarin, and furosemide.

Incontinence Medication Case (Myrbetriq – mirabegron)

An 88 year old female was struggling with incontinence. Upon a nursing assessment, this patient was frequently incontinent throughout the day and night. For her CHF, the patient needed increased doses of diuretics which obviously can make things more problematic by increasing the amount of fluid into the bladder and ultimately increase urine produced. This patient was tried on oxybutynin (Ditropan) with no particular benefit and then transitioned to tolterodine (Detrol). Neither was very effective in improving incontinence, so they were both discontinued.

Mirabegron (Myrbetriq) is a first in class medication that has beta-agonist activity. What does this mean? Beta-blockers (antagonists) are used clinically to lower blood pressure and pulse. An agonist will have the opposite effects. In this case, the Myrbetriq was started and within a few weeks to a couple of months, a noted uptick in blood pressure occurred, resulting in an increase of losartan and amlodipine. Incontinence was not improved enough to make a difference in this case. With the possible side effect of increased BP and zero to minimal effect on incontinence, the risks outweighed the benefits and Myrbetriq was discontinued.

Drug Induced Insomnia/Anxiety

I had a patient who was rehabbing a knee replacement and having some difficulty sleeping. Pain was an important factor to consider, but appeared to be pretty well managed and eventually determined to not be playing a major role in this case. I had discussed the case with nursing, and they stated that he was up all day and all night and did have some anxiety, but he was more concerned that he couldn't sleep. Nursing was questioning if we could try some lorazepam (Ativan) to help with this problem. I said I'd take a look and see what I could figure out. I did not anticipate when reviewing the medication list that the patient would be on a stimulant type medication. This patient was taking modafinil (Provigil) for an unknown reason. I suspect it was maybe to help stimulate energy for rehab as I have seen this off label a couple of different times. Always, always, always look for a drug related reason for the symptoms a patient is experiencing! The modafinil was discontinued, sleep patterns improved, and the unnecessary use of lorazepam to treat side effects of the modafinil was avoided.

Ibuprofen Side Effects: Edema

A 68 year old male battling some knee pain tries ibuprofen 400 mg three times daily to help with osteoarthritis and muscle pain. This gentleman has a history of cardiac issues including CHF and a recent heart attack. He is currently on a low dose of furosemide (Lasix) 20 mg daily for his heart failure and history of edema. He had talked to a neighbor who stated that he uses ibuprofen 800 mg three times daily. Following his neighbor's suggestion, he increases his dose to what his neighbor is taking. Within a couple weeks, his symptoms of edema and CHF dramatically worsened, requiring an increase in furosemide.

Upon questioning, he forgets to tell his provider that he is taking the ibuprofen which can cause side effects like edema. This is another classic example of the prescribing cascade where a new medication causes the addition or increase of another. NSAIDs like ibuprofen can certainly exacerbate CHF.

Another critical aspect of this case is patient education and appropriate assessment of all potential medications. Patients often forget, overlook, or don't recognize the fact that over the counter or herbal medications can cause problems just like prescription medications.

Love the book? If so, please do me a huge favor and leave a kind review on Amazon!

Looking for more content?

Free 6 page PDF – 30 Medication Mistakes - https://www.meded101.com/free-webinar/

Facebook – facebook.com/meded101 -

2 daily medication quiz questions

Twitter – @mededucation101 -
https://twitter.com/Mededucation101

LinkedIn – Connect with me!
Eric Christianson, Pharm.D., BCPS, CGP